compaired to mendel 44

Times, Places, and Persons

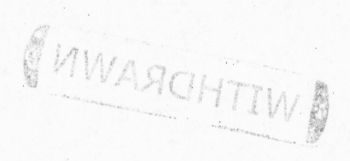

The Henry E. Sigerist Supplements to the
Bulletin of the History of Medicine
New Series, no. 4

Editor: Lloyd G. Stevenson, M.D.

Henry E. Sigerist, recruited by William H. Welch to be director of the Johns Hopkins Institute of the History of Medicine, was the founder of the *Bulletin of the History of Medicine* and also of the first series of supplements, which extended from 1943 to 1951. It was Sigerist's resolve that the *Bulletin* should provide the organ not only of the Johns Hopkins Institute but also the American Association, and to this day it subserves both functions. It is therefore eminently suitable that the new series should bear the founder's name and perpetuate his scholarly interests. These interests were so broad and so varied that the supplements will recognize no narrow limits in range of theme and will publish historical essays of greater scope than the *Bulletin* itself can accommodate. It is not too much to hope that in time the Sigerist supplements will help to extend the purview of medical history.

Other Books in the New Series

1. *Almost Persuaded: American Physicians and Compulsory Health Insurance, 1912-1920*
   by Ronald L. Numbers
2. *William Harvey and His Age: The Professional and Social Context of the Discovery of the Circulation*
   edited by Jerome J. Bylebyl
3. *The Clinical Training of Doctors: An Essay of 1793*
   by Philippe Pinel
   edited and translated, with an introductory essay, by Dora B. Weiner

A Conference on the History of Epidemiology
Sponsored by
The Josiah Macy, Jr. Foundation
and
The Johns Hopkins University
Institute of the History of Medicine and
School of Hygiene and Public Health
May 5, 1978

TIMES, PLACES, AND PERSONS

ASPECTS OF THE HISTORY OF EPIDEMIOLOGY

Edited by
Abraham M. Lilienfeld, M.D.

THE JOHNS HOPKINS UNIVERSITY PRESS
BALTIMORE AND LONDON

This book has been brought to publication with the generous assistance of the Josiah Macy, Jr. Foundation.

The Johns Hopkins University Press, Baltimore, Maryland 21218
The Johns Hopkins Press Ltd., London

Library of Congress Cataloging in Publication Data

Conference on the History of Epidemiology, Johns
    Hopkins University, 1978.
    Times, places, and persons.

    (The Henry E. Sigerist supplements to the Bulletin
of the history of medicine; new ser., no. 4)
    Presented by the Johns Hopkins University Institute
of the History of Medicine and School of Hygiene and
Public Health.
    Includes bibliographical references and index.
    1. Epidemiology—History—Congresses.
I. Lilienfeld, Abraham M. II. Johns Hopkins University.
Institute of the History of Medicine.
III. Johns Hopkins University. School of Hygiene and
Public Health. IV. Title. V. Series: Henry E.
Sigerist supplements to the Bulletin of the history
of medicine; new ser., no. 4.
RA649.C66 1978   614.4'09   80-8090
ISBN 0-8018-2425-7 (pbk.)

Contents

Preface

The marked growth of epidemiology as a scientific discipline is evident in its widening scope of application to the entire range of public health and medical problems. Paralleling this growth, epidemiology has also matured in its methodologic and inferential content. A sign of such maturation is the increased interest in the historical background and development of epidemiology by its practitioners as well as its historians. Thus, the time was ripe for organizing this Conference on the History of Epidemiology which was presented on May 5, 1978, by The Johns Hopkins University, Institute of the History of Medicine and School of Hygiene and Public Health, with the generous support of the Josiah Macy, Jr. Foundation.

In planning the Conference, it was recognized that the perceptions of historians and of epidemiologists do differ. The historian takes into consideration the total historical context within which a discipline develops, whereas the epidemiologist is usually more concerned with its internal conceptual changes. Consequently, it was considered desirable to intermesh these two aspects to the largest extent possible. In an attempt to achieve this objective, it was arranged to have a historian discuss an epidemiologist's presentation and conversely to have an epidemiologist discuss a historian's presentation. In addition, the president of each of the professional organizations of these two disciplines, the American Epidemiological Society and the American Association for the History of Medicine, chaired the morning and afternoon sessions, respectively.

Modern epidemiology essentially originated in the beginning of the nineteenth century with William Farr as one of its leaders and with the French hygienic movement playing a major role; the conceptual origins and contributions of Farr are discussed by Eyler and that of the hygienic movement by the Lilienfelds. Today, close relationships exist between the fields of statistics and epidemiology. This was historically always true, as shown by Hilts's review of the statistical movement of the nineteenth century and its relationship to epidemiologic thinking.

ix

After this general background is painted on the historical canvas, more specific areas are reviewed, with Roe first summarizing the various attempts at eradicating pellagra. This is followed by a consideration of infectious diseases, where epidemiology has made major contributions to their understanding and control. First, Richmond reviews the conceptual history of the germ theory of disease. Then Henderson's presentation of the history of the eradication of smallpox brings us to the contemporary scene. Finally Woodward discusses yellow fever, a disease yet to be conquered.

The formal discussions of each of these presentations are included in this volume. With these, new issues and questions are raised, clearly indicating that the Conference represents only the beginning of this historical quest.

Times, Places, and Persons

The Conceptual Origins
of William Farr's Epidemiology:
Numerical Methods and Social Thought in the 1830s

John M. Eyler

British and American epidemiologists looking for the historical roots of their discipline have assigned unusual importance to William Farr. According to Sir Arthur Newsholme, "Farr must be ranked with William Harvey in Physiology or with Lavoisier in chemistry . . . [He] was a chief architect of the public health administration, which during his life-time was built up chiefly by three men, Edwin Chadwick, John Simon, and Farr himself."[1] Writing nearly a quarter-century later, Major Greenwood expressed similar views. The methods of using vital data which Farr introduced were "the most valuable single instrument of social-medical research our national armoury contains."[2] More recently Alexander Langmuir and the Lilienfelds have written enthusiastic appreciations of Farr's epidemiological work, dwelling on both concept and method.[3] In the new introduction to the recent republication of Farr's memorial volume we read that Farr was "a founder, even the founder, of epidemiology in its modern form."[4] The authors of this introduction, Mervyn Susser and Abraham Adelstein, point out that Farr developed tools that have stood the test of time: a standard nosology, standardized death rates, and mathematical models for complex epidemiological phenomena such as the curve of an epidemic or the relationship between population density and mortality.

In explaining Farr's success and influence in epidemiology much importance must be assigned to the favorable circumstances in which he worked. He was the first statistical heir of the newly created system of civil registration. As the chief statistician of England's General Register Office he inherited a wealth of vital data unknown to previous statisticians. Over his forty-year civil service career he commanded the civil registration system and for part of that time the statistical services of the

1

census as well. Much of his energy went into devising ways to organize and exploit this factual harvest. In this work he had the aid of a staff of trained clerks and eventually of a primitive computer, a model of a Babbage calculator.[5] With this statistical organization behind him Farr was able to bring to the problems he chose unprecedented quantities of statistical information, information collected year after year in a uniform manner; thus in the realm of vital statistics he spoke with unrivaled authority. But as important as this newly available data was and as essential as the devices Farr devised to handle it became, these facts do not in themselves entirely explain his success. Even before civil registration began we find important suggestions and novel departures in the writings of young Farr, then a struggling general practitioner and medical journalist.[6]

The main thesis of this paper can be stated briefly. Farr's basic ideas coalesced in the middle 1830s. By the time he joined the General Register Office full time in 1839 he had formed the conceptual framework around which his later statistical and epidemiological work was fashioned. The key components of Farr's synthesis were: first, a firm commitment to environmental reform in which political and medical ideals reinforced each other; second, a belief that statistics offered the hope of advancing both social progress and medical knowledge; and third, the imaginative use of a fruitful numerical approach Farr discovered in the work of a comparatively unknown British actuary.

Farr was one of many professional-class men who were profoundly affected by the Reform Movement. He was twenty-nine years old and still a student when the Reform Bill became law. As a young general practitioner he watched with much interest the passage of the New Poor Law, the Factory Act, the Municipal Corporations Act, and of course the Registration Act. Behind this political reform and social legislation lay deep concerns about the social order and the stability of established institutions. At the root of this anxiety lay the problem of poverty and the condition of the urban working class.

Recent historical scholarship has shown an ambivalence or tension in the thought of middle class reformers in this decade between on the one hand, a moralistic interpretation of poverty which blamed the poor for their own misery and opposed public intervention on their behalf, and on the other hand, an environmentalist interpretation which explained suffering and moral failure as the products of miserable conditions of life and sought solutions in public action.[7] Farr shared this ambivalence. The editorials for the medical journal he published in

1837, *British Annals of Medicine, Pharmacy, Vital Statistics,* and *General Science,* show no sympathy for "the idle, reckless, vicious . . ." or "the worthless hereditary vagabond."[8] But on the other hand Farr had a genuine sympathy for the worthy poor, an empathy that sprang perhaps from his own humble origins.[9] Relief of poverty and distress was necessary, at least temporarily, to protect innocent life as well as to stabilize the social order. But according to Farr, again in 1837, the punitive welfare scheme masterminded by Edwin Chadwick was an embarrassment to right-thinking men.

We believe it now to be a prevalent opinion, among the majority of reflecting men, that the grand object of every good government should be to protect the weak from the tyranny or oppression of the more powerful. . . . Even under our reform government, we blush to say that the poor—the weak—who are always least able to defend themselves, have been, in the case of the New Poor-law, very harshily dealth with.[10]

Despite the complexity of Farr's views about the nature and causes of human misery, he generally concluded that public intervention was part of the solution. The state must act. The purpose of its intervention was not paternal care and, consequently, dependency, but it was the provision of the prerequisites for social advancement through the efforts of the poor themselves.[11] Chief among those necessary preconditions was human health.

Current trends in medical thinking about the nature and causes of disease encouraged Farr to equate health and social condition. It was common knowledge that certain epidemic and endemic diseases accompanied human misery. With the decline of the doctrine of contagion during the twenties and thirties in the face of medical experience with typhus, observations on tropical diseases, and the failure of quarantine during the first pandemic of Asiatic cholera, medical men gave renewed attention to conditions which were believed to generate diseases locally. Farr worked out a very sensible compromise on this complex question.[12] In his own disease theory he preserved a small role for contagion and a larger role for specific, disease-causing materials. His major attention was devoted, however, to environmental conditions, particularly poor sanitation and overcrowding, which, he believed, favored both the spread and also the generation of disease.

Farr could reason then on credible evidence that the living conditions of the urban poor were responsible for the notorious insalubrity of large cities. He also adopted the more extreme position of using the prevalence of preventable disease as a form of social criticism.[13] "For death is the exponent of misery," he explained in 1837.[14] Two years later he referred to diseases as "the iron index of misery."[15] Nearly three decades later we find him claiming: "No variation in the health of the states of Europe is the result of chance; it is the direct result of the physical and political conditions in which nations live."[16] In the 1870s he argued that there were relationships not only between death and health, sickness, mental energy, and "national primacy," but also between the forms of death and "moral excellence or infamy:"[17]

It is clear then why Farr's commitment to sanitary reform was intense. It came from both sentiment—from the desire to save innocent lives—and from a conviction that sanitary reform was essential to save Western industrial society from political disaster. It is little wonder then that he regarded the investigation of the causes of disease and premature death and the development of policies of prevention as the most worthy subjects of endeavor. It is also not surprising that he was unable to compromise on final goals or that in describing them he often resorted to intense, emotionally charged rhetoric that his more narrow-minded colleagues in later decades found disquieting.[18]

In the Thirties Farr's reform impulses found more professional focuses as well. He joined a group of extreme advocates of medical reform who constituted the first and short-lived British Medical Association.[19] In a series of editorials and in a reform oration to his colleagues Farr roundly condemned the medical establishment for governing the profession in ways out of harmony with the democratic aspirations of the age and for intellectual incompetence resulting from an ignorance of recent advances in the sciences.[20] Farr believed the reforms he advocated were the counterpart of the political and social reforms underway, and he freely used liberal reform rhetoric in making his case.

Granting then Farr's reformist sympathies, we may still wonder why should he have turned to statistics. Actually, in the early Victorian period the choice was a fairly natural one. Popular interest in statistics in the Thirties was very high.[21] In a flourish of activity statistical societies were founded in London and in several provincial cities. This statistical movement was itself a product of the broader reform movement. The founders of the statistical societies were members of the commercial and professional classes who saw in the use of social facts a valuable weapon for the reform cause. Statistics, these men believed, was a science, but they did not conceive of it as a mathematical science (indeed few of the founding members had mastered more mathematics than shop arithmetic). They thought of statistics rather as a social science, as the science of social reform.[22] This vision of statistics had great appeal. A new science, so conceived, gave reform sympathies a focus and a program. It promised to defuse party passion and to substitute for rhetoric, certainty based upon the accumulation of irrefutable facts. According to the ideals of that period the science of statistics would discover the principles of legislation and administration. It would make social reform certain or "scientific." What the founders apparently wanted above all was to make reform safe, to find a way of protecting cherished institutions while advocating a limited range of social reforms, mainly educational and sanitary.[23]

Medical men like Farr had a special interest in statistics and in the statistical societies. Sympathies with the reform movement led many doctors to the statistical societies. James Phillips Kay, later Kay-Shuttleworth, is only the best known of many physicians who helped found and direct the early provincial statistical societies.[24] Progressive medical men had special reasons for taking up statistics. Voices in the profession were then proclaiming that statistics, or the Numerical Method, promised to provide the tool to advance medical knowledge. William Guy made this claim in a well-known paper to the Statistical Society of London and so did several other authors who relied on Guy: Doctors Daniel and William Griffin and an anonymous author in the *British and Foreign Medical Review* who discussed Jules Gavarret's work on medical statistics.[25] These men argued that in order to improve itself medicine must emulate the methods of the physical sciences. In particular, physicians must learn to make precise measurements and to use quantitative methods. In an effective section the Griffins compared the "irregularity, uncertainty, and confusion" of medicine whose practitioners relied on memory for facts, used such terms as "generally, not unfrequently, sometimes," and quarreled among themselves on even the fundamentals of their discipline, with the precision, the theoretical harmony, and the success in prediction of the physical sciences.[26] They suggested that if physicians would adopt the use of statistics they would improve both prognostics and therapeutics and also discover the causes of disease.

The idea was extremely attractive and the analogy of the higher sciences probably convincing. But there is one glaring fault with these tracts. Behind the glowing optimism was a nearly complete absence of concrete, practical suggestions. Medicine should employ numbers, but how? The Griffins and the British reviewer of Gavarret's work mention Pierre Louis's studies but criticize them for methodological weaknesses.[27]

Guy pointed to Quetelet's work to establish that complex human events, even those involving the will, when observed in the aggregate, exhibit similar law-abiding tendencies.[28] But there was little specific guidance in these tracts for practitioners. The suggestions of these proponents of the Numerical Method in Britain seem to reduce themselves to little more than this: Collect and arrange all the measurements you can; once you have found your averages, we can tell you how to calculate their limits of error.[29]

Farr was one of few men in early Victorian England to discover fruitful ways of applying numerical analysis to the health problems of interest to the medical reformers. This discovery came early in his career, immediately prior to the publishing of the tracts just mentioned.[30] The origins of the specific quantitative techniques Farr developed can, I believe, be traced to the publications in the early and middle Thirties of the British actuary, Thomas Rowe Edmonds. Edmonds published a work on life tables in 1832 in which he announced an important discovery, that human mortality was geometrically related to human age.[31] More specifically, Edmonds found that the mortality figures for consecutive ages from the best available life tables formed three geometrical series, for the years before, during, and after the period of procreative power. From six weeks of age until six to nine years the mortality dropped 32.4% each year. From then until puberty mortality was at its lowest. During the period of procreative power, mortality increased annually at 2.991%. After the period of procreative power mortality increased much faster, at an annual rate of 7.969%. Edmonds called this discovery the law of mortality. Previous actuaries had used the phrase but not with precisely this meaning. Edmonds believed it was a general law expressing some fundamental feature of human biology. Absolute mortality might differ between two populations and so might the precise limits of the period of procreative power, but the pattern of change of mortality with age was universal.

Edmonds suggested this fact made it possible to compute, by extrapolation, theoretical life tables that would be more uniform and accurate than tables drawn exclusively from experience. In figure 1 we see him comparing mortality rates from three such theoretical tables with rates from commonly used experiential tables. His Village Mortality Table, which had been formed by assuming a mortality of five per thousand at the age of ten and then applying his law, agreed well with Joshua Milne's Carlisle Table. The Mean Mortality Table, which was generated by assuming a mortality of six per thousand at age ten, agreed closely with

Between Ages.	Six Towns of England.	Glasgow.	London.	Theoretical Tables.			Sweden, 21 years, 1755-75.	England and Wales.	Carlisle, 9 Years, 1779-87.
				City Mortality.	Mean Mortality.	Village Mortality.			
0— 5	8.63	8.10	8.27	8.46	6.73	7.48	9.01	4.98	8.23
5—10	1.03	1.24	1.08	1.24	.99	1.02	1.42	.70	1.02
10—20	.73	.76	.60	.88	.70	.58	.71	.63	.59
20—30	1.39	1.17	1.07	1.17	.93	.78	.92	1.02	.75
30—40	1.56	1.57	1.52	1.57	1.25	1.05	1.22	1.19	1.06
40—50	1.96	2.31	2.29	2.10	1.68	1.40	1.74	1.49	1.43
50—60	3.00	3.50	3.61	2.99	2.40	2.01	2.64	2.25	1.83
60—70	5.83	6.04	7.34	5.99	4.83	4.05	4.81	4.33	4.12
70—80	12.10	13.57	15.23	12.36	10.04	8.46	10.23	9.90	8.30
80—90	24.62	23.81	29.91	24.53	20.18	17.16	20.78	22.08	17.56
Above 90	42.72	42.55	33.55	47.20	39.85	33.45	39.41	37.10	28.44
All ages	2.95	2.83	2.84	—	—	—	2.89	2.12	2.50

FIGURE 1. Comparison of age-group mortality rates from theoretical and experiential life tables. T.R. Edmonds, "On the mortality at Glasgow, and on the increasing mortality in England," *Lancet,* 1835-36, *2:* 358.

the table Richard Price had computed from Swedish data. His City Mortality Table assumed the mortality at age ten was 7.5 per thousand and agree well with the best available data for large British cities. This technique of comparing a theoretical series, generated by a formula, and a series of observations is one Edmonds frequently used.

Edmonds' law was not as original as its author believed. He in fact had independently discovered the relationship Benjamin Gompertz announced to the Royal Society of London in 1825.[32] For the purposes we are considering, Edmonds' formulation had several advantages. His derivation was mathematically simpler than that of Gompertz. Further-more, Edmonds made an effort to bring his discovery to the attention of the medical profession. In a series of articles in *The Lancet* for 1835 through 1837 Edmonds explained in very simple terms his discovery, and suggested several ways in which it could be used to study human health and disease.[33]

Edmonds' discovery of this law of human mortality and his sugges-tions about its applications made a deep impression on Farr. Farr's *British Medical Almanack* carried a summary article by Edmonds, and in Farr's first comprehensive article on vital statistics there are repeated references to Edmonds.[34] At the most formal level we can see that Farr adopted Edmonds' suggestion on using extensive interpolative techniques

Between Ages	Relative Sickness and Death.					Absolute number constantly Sick, & dying annually, out of 100 living.			
	20-30	30-40	40-50	50-60	Common Multiplier	20-30	30-40	40-50	50-60
Sickness { Scotland	.57	.67	1.00	1.83	1.97	1.13	1.32	1.97	3.60
England	.60	.71	1.00	1.69	2.56	1.54	1.83	2.56	4.32
Deaths ... England	.51	.78	1.00	1.61	1.85	.95	1.45	1.85	2.98
Theory	.55	.74	1.00	1.43	—	—	—	—	—

FIGURE 2. Theoretical and observed series for sickness and death by age. T.R. Edmonds, "On the laws of sickness, according to age . . . ," *Lancet*, 1835-36, *1:* 856.

to construct life tables by assuming that mortality changed regularly with age over several periods of life.[35] But Edmonds' example was even more important as an inspiration for approaches and methods. Farr recognized that what Edmonds had done for the general law of mortality in a life table might be done for other vital phenomena: that is, one might show mutual relationships by discovering that observations formed a series or several related series which could be described mathematically. In doing this, one gained that power of the higher sciences medical men of this generation so prized, the power of prediction. Edmonds' work thus confirmed Farr's belief that vital phenomena were law-abiding, and it suggested a method. Farr began to seek statistical laws of the sort Edmonds had discovered and he demonstrated these laws by comparing a computed and an observed series. He also occasionally tried to predict future events by extending a theoretical series.

Edmonds had made several suggestions that probably encouraged Farr to consider certain statistical applications. In his series of articles in *The Lancet* Edmonds had suggested that the law of mortality also applied to sickness.[36] More specifically, he found in limited data from Friendly Societies and from the London Fever Hospital that both the number of cases of sickness and the case fatality from one disease, fever, increased with each year of age—at least during the middle years of life—at the same rate as the general mortality of the population (figures 2 and 3). He suggested that this discovery might be used to judge the effectiveness of therapy.

Edmonds' suggestion seems to have inspired Farr's most remarkable early study, three articles in which he proposed a system he called "nosometry" for bringing statistics to the aid of clinical judgment.[37] Using the records of nearly five thousand cases of smallpox for patients

Between Ages.	Out of 100 attacked by Fever, there die according to	
	Fact.	Theory.
5—16	8.3	—
15—26	11.5	12.5
25—36	17.1	16.8
35—46	22.0	22.6
45—56	30.5	30.3
55—66	40.7	40.7
Above 65	44.6	—

FIGURE 3. Theoretical and observed case fatality rates by age, *Ibid.*, 858.

aged ten to thirty-five years who had been treated at the London Small-pox Hospital, Farr constructed a sickness table (fig. 4). For each consecutive five-day period from the fifth to the one hundred and fifth day, the table displayed the number dying, the number recovering, and the number who remained sick from a cohort of 10,000. The table was in fact analogous to a life table, except that instead of two basic columns, the living and the dying, it had three: the sick, the recovering, and the dying. From the table one could easily see the way in which the chances of recovery or of death changed during the course of disease. Farr discovered two statistical laws at work in this table, one for mortality in smallpox and a complementary one for recovery (fig. 5).

Farr suggested that the construction and application of sickness tables would do much to improve the practice of medicine. With such tables before him, a practitioner could determine for any period of the disease, the likelihood of recovery and the probable future duration of the case. Prognosis would thus be made much more accurate as well as easier. Furthermore, with the use of such tables the effectiveness of therapy could be objectively determined. Comparison of tables for the same disease treated by different regimens would show clearly which regimen either increased the chances of recovery or shortened the duration of cases.

Farr's nosometry is thus an amazing methodological suggestion for the 1830s. Judged exclusively as a statistical tool it was superior to the

Day	Sick	To Recover	To Die	Terminating	Recovering	Dying	Day
	A	B	C	D	E	F	
0	—	-	-	-	-	-	0
5	10000	6589	3411	317	-	317	5
10	9683	6589	3094	1370	46	1324	10
15	8313	6543	1770	1185	54	1131	15
20	7128	6489	639	578	265	313	20
25	6550	6224	326	769	639	130	25
30	5781	5585	196	976	898	78	30
35	4805	4687	118	1055	1008	47	35
40	3750	3679	71	922	894	28	40
45	2828	2785	43	694	677	17	45
50	2134	2108	26	515	513	2	50
55	1619	1595	24	390	388	2	55
60	1229	1207	22	295	293	2	60
65	934	914	20	225	223	2	65
70	709	691	18	170	168	2	70
75	539	523	16	129	127	2	75
80	410	396	14	98	96	2	80
85	312	300	12	75	73	2	85
90	237	227	10	57	55	2	90
95	180	172	8	44	42	2	95
100	136	130	6	34	32	2	100
105	102	98	4	-	-	-	105
-	400	400	2	-	-	-	-

FIGURE 4. Sickness table for smallpox. W[illiam] Farr, "On a method of determining the danger and the duration of diseases at every period of their progress," *Brit. Ann. Med.*, 1837, *1:* 76.

Day	To Recover.		To Die.	
	Theory.	Fact.	Fact.	Theory.
0				
5	3314	3314	1601	1601
10	3314	3314	1452	1452
15	3291	3296	821	831
20	3263	3268	300	300
25	3130	3117	153	153
30	2809	2817	92	92
35	2357	2360	54	55
40	1850	1848	33	33
45	1400	1406	21	20
50	1060	1039	13	12
55	802	804	12	11
60	607			10
65	459	450	9	9
70	348			8
75	264	280	7	7

FIGURE 5. Observed and calculated series for recoveries and deaths in smallpox. *Ibid.*, 75.

DEATHS observed in the decline of the Epidemic.

1	2	3	4	5	6	7
4365	4087	3767	3416	2743	2019	1631

DEATHS in a regular series.

1	2	3	4	5	6	7
4364	4147	3767	3272	2716	2156	1635

FIGURE 6. Observed and calculated series of smallpox deaths describing the fall of an epidemic. Farr, "Letter," *2nd A.R.R.G.,* p. 96 [B.P.P., 1840, XVII, p. 19].

methods Pierre Louis was then using in Paris. It was infinitely superior to the attempts of certain of Farr's immediate British predecessors. In the latter category are Sir Gilbert Blane and F. Bisset Hawkins, both of whom attempted to vindicate contemporary therapy for acute diseases by comparing the success of modern physicians with that of the Hippocratic physicians recorded in *Epidemics I* and *III.*[38] The success of the latter was taken to represent the outcome of the cases left to the healing power of nature.

Farr's nosometry seems to have found no serious imitators in England. Although Farr repeated his suggestion years later, in 1862,[39] his attention had shifted to epidemiological problems by 1840. However, the basic drive to discover statistical laws of the sort Edmonds brought to his attention remained with him and encouraged Farr to try to describe statistically the course of an epidemic. An epidemic of smallpox was in progress when civil registration began. After ten quarters of registration Farr showed that the number of smallpox deaths for the nation as a whole and for certain smaller geographical regions was falling in a manner he could describe by a geometric series (fig. 6).[40] Like Edmonds, Farr worked by subtracting one or more orders of the differences of logarithms. Perhaps for this reason he missed the fact that his figures for the Metropolis conformed to Quetelet's law of error (fig. 7).

The fact that epidemics could be described by geometric series suggested the possibility of predicting their future course. Farr was not slow to exploit this potential. When smallpox deaths again began to climb in the Metropolis, Farr showed that if he had used the rate of increase for the previous epidemic to predict the course of the present he would not have been far from the mark (fig. 8).[41] His boldest prediction came not from the study of human disease, but in his response to Robert Lowe's gloomy prognostication about the outcome of rinderpest or Cattle Plague.[42] On the basis of only four quarterly returns Farr predicted that

(n) SMALL-POX.

Years	1837		1838				1839			
Periods	1	2	3	4	5	6	7	8	9	10
Liverpool and West Derby .	458	176	52	33	18	37	13	34	75	141
Manchester. .	23	98	127	120	111	180	94	40	33	53
Bath . . .	154	18	15	1	1	2	1	25	17	30
Exeter . . .	88	131	6	..	2	..	..	..	..	..
Leeds . . .	4	11	29	69	134	197	74	55	30	15
Norwich . .	1	..	..	..	..	17	180	204	10	7
Metropolis . .	257	506	753	1145	1061	858	364	117	63	60

FIGURE 7. Quarterly smallpox deaths in London 1837-1839. *Ibid.*, 92 [16].

DEATHS BY SMALL-POX.

	Registered.	Series of Numbers produced by 1 65, the Rate of Increase in the Epidemic of 1837-8.
13 weeks (Oct. 1 to Dec. 31, 1839).....	60	60
13 weeks (Jan. 5 to April 4, 1840)......	104	99
13 weeks (April 5 to July 4)	170	163
13 weeks (July 5 to Oct. 3)............	253	267
Total.....................	587	589

FIGURE 8. Observed and calculated series describing rise of smallpox epidemic. William Farr, "Note on the present epidemic of smallpox, and on the necessity of arresting its ravages," *Lancet*, 1840-41, *1:* 352.

the epidemic was about to subside. It was an extremely bold prediction because he had to assume that the third order difference of consecutive logarithms for the series were constant. With only four figures he, of course, had only one third order difference. Figure 9 is a comparison John Brownlee published in 1915 of the recorded fatalities from rinderpest and of Farr's calculated series. Such a prediction indicates an extreme faith in the lawfulness of the progress of epidemics.

It is possible to trace the development of this approach to several of Farr's major studies in which he tried to demonstrate the influence of

Periods of Four Weeks ending			Reported Attacks.	Calculated Series by "Law."	Actual Figures.*
1865 -					
November 4	...	...	9,597	9,597	9,597
December 2	...	...	18,817	18,817	18,817
December 30	...	...	33,835	33,835	33,835
1866 -					
January 27...	...	...	47,191	47,191	47,287
February 24	...	...		43,182	57,004
March 24	...	...	...	21,927	27,958
April 21	...	...	...	5,226	15,856
May 19	...	...	...	494	14,734
June 16	...	...	...	16	5,000 (about)

FIGURE 9. The course of the cattle plague (1865-1866) and Farr's prediction. John Brownlee, "Historical note on Farr's theory of the epidemic," *Brit. J. Med.*, 1915, *2:* 251.

the environment on human mortality. The numerical methods he employed in these cases no longer show a strong resemblance to those Edmonds used, but they can be regarded as later elaborations of ideas that Edmonds' work had suggested to Farr in the 1830s. Farr's law of elevation for the London cholera epidemic of 1849 may be regarded in this light.[43] What this law established was that the cholera mortality in the registration districts of the Metropolis was inversely related to the mean elevation of those districts above the high water mark of the Thames. The relationship was suggested by his disease theory. He proved it by showing that the series of mortality rates for the districts in consecutive twenty foot terraces above the Thames could be approximated by a theoretical series. Figure 10 shows Farr's observed and calculated series as he presented them. Figure 11 presents curves Langmuir drew to illustrate the agreement between the two sets of figures.

Farr faced a similar problem in trying to prove that human mortality increased with population density. This was a relationship which both his disease theory and his reform ideas encouraged him to believe existed. But in spite of several attempts he had been unable to find a satisfying numerical expression for it.[44] At the very end of his career he showed that there was a numerical relationship between mortality of mean duration of life and mean proximity, the latter being defined as the

Mean Elevation of the ground above the High-water Mark.	Mean Mortality from Cholera.	Calculated Series.
0	177	174
10	102	99
30	65	53
50	34	34
70	27	27
90	22	22
100	17	20
—	—	—
350	7	6

FIGURE 10. Observed and calculated series for Farr's elevation law for cholera. [William Farr], *Report on the Mortality of Cholera in England, 1848-49* (London, 1952), p. lxiii.

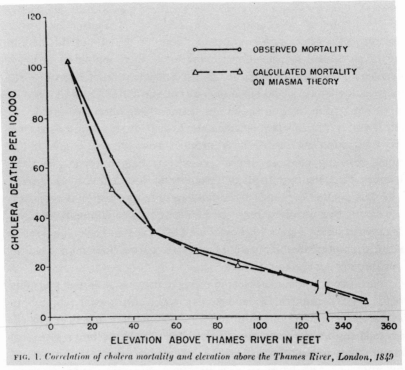

FIG. 1. *Correlation of cholera mortality and elevation above the Thames River, London, 1849*

FIGURE 11. Graphical representation of the two series in illustration seven. Alexander D. Langmuir, "Epidemiology of airborne infection," *Bact. Rev.* 25 (1961), 174.

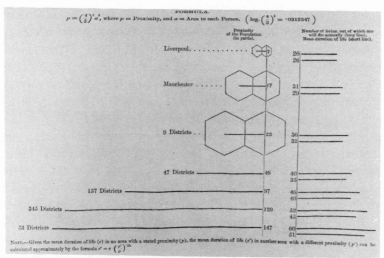

FIGURE 12. Farr's diagram illustrating his law for the relation of mortality to proximity of population. Farr, "Letter," *40th A.R.R.G.,* p. 237 [B.P.P., 1878-79, XIX].

distance between the centers of coterminous regular hexagons which represented each resident's share of territory if the land of the district were to be equally divided (fig. 12).[45] Farr's formula allowed him to compute the mean duration of life or the mortality of one district if he knew its proximity and both the proximity and mean duration of life or the mortality of a second district. Arithmetically the law was only one step removed from the elevation law for cholera.

There is a second area in which Edmonds' work of the Thirties may have had a formative influence on Farr. Edmonds had suggested that life tables might be used as a measure of health and vitality. Using census materials, in particular the voluntary returns of the ages of the living for the 1821 census and the retrospective returns of the ages of the deaths from the parish registers for the 1831 census (1813-1830), Edmonds constructed life tables for the entire population and for the residents of certain geographical areas such as counties.[46] He compared mortality rates from these tables to illustrate the differences in health of the people, and he cautioned that differences in age composition of populations made comparisons of crude mortality rates untrustworthy. In these articles he compared mortality rates for broad age groups for the counties of England and suggested that the mortality of females aged 15 to 60 was probably the best comparative index of health.[47]

Edmonds' appreciation of the important effect that the age composition of the population had on its crude mortality rate was not novel in actuarial circles, but it was an effect that was not well understood among the general public or in the medical profession. Perhaps because of Edmonds' warnings, Farr, from the very beginning of his career, appreciated the hazards of comparing crude mortality rates. In his finest studies Farr used life tables, or more properly, life table death rates, as the measure of health. We can see this approach in his study of the health of large towns. The focus of his first reports to the Registrar General was an attempt to demonstrate the extent to which health deteriorates in the environment of large cities. In the first three of these reports he simply compared the total number of deaths and the deaths from certain causes in the Metropolis and in a group of rural districts from the south of England which had a combined population equal to that of the Metropolis.[48] But in the fifth report he was able to use the returns of the living for the 1841 census and the registration returns of death for the same year to construct life tables for the nation as a whole and for three areas which represented England's range of salubrity: rural Surrey, the Metropolis, and Liverpool.[49] Figures 13 and 14 are Farr's illustrations of the results. The white area represents the number of the living and the black area the number of deaths in a cohort of 100,000. Using these tables Farr estimated the number of preventable deaths in the Metropolis and in Liverpool. As a means of comparing the health of places, his method was a distinct improvement over his previous efforts, which were in effect comparisons of crude mortality rates, and over Edwin Chadwick's controversial comparisons of the mean age at death in districts.[50]

Farr continued to refine the use of life tables as comparative measures of health. In the 1860s he again tried to show the unnecessary loss of life which occurred in British cities. He now compared the experience of the residents of England's thirty large towns with that of a standard population, the residents of the Healthy Districts. By applying the age-specific mortality rates from his Healthy District Life Table to the urban population alive in each of the same age groups, he was able to show what the mortality of the large towns would have been, had they been subjected to the same law of mortality as the standard population (fig. 15).[51] In more contemporary terms, he had begun to compare standardized death rates.

The purpose of this discussion has been to identify the essential components in the formation of Farr's epidemiological concepts. We have tried to suggest that there is a continuity of numerical methods in Farr's major studies which can be traced ultimately to suggestions Farr

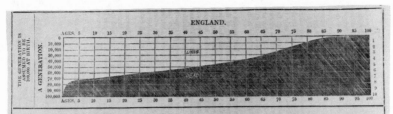

"The first diagram is intended to represent the progress of an English generation through life the light part indicating the living, the dark the dead, at each age out of a given number (100,000) born alive. The vertical lines divided into ten degrees serve to measure, at every fifth year, the number alive and dead at the respective ages. The areas of the enclosed light spaces serve also to show the relative numbers living. The second, third, and fourth, diagrams exhibit the same facts for Surrey, Liverpool, and the Metropolis. The extent of light space upon each diagram gives a general notion of the relative population which would be maintained in the different circumstances by an *equal number* of births; but this is more clearly seen in the second set of diagrams (p. 52), in which the light space representing the living is thrown into the form of parallelograms. These parallelograms are divided by vertical lines, so as to show the relative numbers that would be living at the different ages (if the births were not more than the deaths) in Surrey, Liverpool, and the Metropolis. At the four very different rates of mortality, such would be the relative population of the kingdom—such the relative numbers of children, adults, and old people, to the same number of births. Observation has, however, shown that the births increase generally as the deaths increase; and the parallelogram of Liverpool, to represent the population of an unhealthy place (into which there was no immigration), must gain in breadth, particularly at the end on the left hand, representing the births, the space which it loses in length."—p. 38.

It will be seen by these Diagrams, that of the 100,000 born alive in Surrey, more than the half (50,000) are alive at the age of 50 ; while out of the same number born alive, 41,000 live to the age of 50 in the Metropolis, and 26,000 in Liverpool.

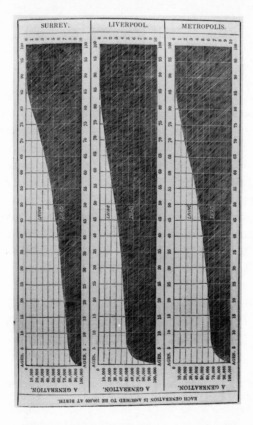

FIGURES 13. and 14. Farr's diagrams comparing the mortality from life tables for England, rural Surrey, Liverpool and the Metropolis. *5th A.R.R.G.*, pp. 50-51 [B.P.P., 1843, XXI, pp. xxxvi-xxxvii].

TABLE XVIII.—**Deaths in 30 Large Town Districts** in the 10 Years 1851–60 ;
and also the DEATHS which would have occurred in the 10 Years if the
MORTALITY had been at the same Rate as prevailed in the 63 HEALTHY DISTRICTS
(1849–53).

AGES.	DEATHS in 10 Years 1851–60.	DEATHS which would have occurred in the 10 Years at HEALTHY DISTRICT RATES.	EXCESS of ACTUAL DEATHS in 10 Years over DEATHS at HEALTHY DISTRICT RATES.
ALL AGES -	711,944	384,590	327,354
0– - -	338,990	135,470	203,520
5– - -	31,319	19,290	12,029
10– - -	14,240	11,020	3,220
15– - -	43,807	37,550	6,257
25– - -	48,625	36,150	12,475
35– - -	50,071	30,320	19,751
45– - -	49,638	26,680	22,958
55– - -	49,763	27,020	22,743
65– - -	47,445	31,510	15,935
75– - -	30,583	22,920	7,663
85 & upwards -	7,463	6,660	803

FIGURE 15. Farr's use ot standardized death rates. Farr, "Letter," *Suppl. 25th A.R.R.G.,*
p. xxvi [B.P.P., 1865, XIII].

discovered in the works of Thomas Rowe Edmonds. While it is undoubtedly true that Farr developed these basic ideas beyond anything
Edmonds had imagined, Edmonds' work was very influential. Farr seems
to have found in it a solution to a problem that troubled reform-minded
British medical men of the 1830s. The problem was to establish a quantitative medical science which would become an engine of reform of both
medical knowledge and social welfare. Farr was deeply committed to
this endeavor. In the 1830s he fashioned statistical tools which he later
used with great imagination to build a program of health surveillance,
research, and public health advocacy. Actuarial methods were a crucial
element in this attempt to translate reform aspirations into professional
action. In the process Farr helped establish procedures and standards
that have survived in twentieth-century epidemiology.

Notes

1. Arthur Newsholme, "William Farr" [a lecture at the Johns Hopkins University, n.d.]
in London School of Economics, Farr Collection, Vol. IX, Item 5, p. 203.

2. Major Greenwood, *Some British Pioneers of Social Medicine* (London: Oxford
University Press, 1948), p. 79.

3. Alexander D. Langmuir, "William Farr: Founder of modern concepts of surveillance,"
Intern. J. Epidemiol., 1976, 5:13-18; and David E. Lilienfeld and Abraham M. Lilienfeld,
"Epidemiology: A retrospective study," *Amer. J. Epidemiol.,* 1977, *106:* 448-449.

4. Mervyn Susser and Abraham Adelstein, "Introduction," *Vital Statistics: A Memorial Volume of Selections from the Reports and Writings of William Farr* [1885] (Metuchen, N.J.: Scarecrow Press, 1975), p. iii. For the following evaluations see also pp. viii and xi-xiii.

5. *English Life Table: Tables of Lifetimes, Annuities, and Premiums,* with an Introduction by William Farr (London, 1864), pp. cxxxix-cxliv.

6. The best biographical account of Farr is still Noel A. Humphreys's Introduction to *Vital Statistics: A Memorial Volume of Selections from the Reports and Writings of William Farr* (London, 1885), pp. vii-xxiv.

7. See for example M.J. Cullen, *The Statistical Movement in Early Victorian Britain: The Foundations of Empirical Social Research* (New York: Barnes & Noble, 1975) esp. pp. 135-146.

8. "Medical relief of paupers," *Brit. Ann. Med.,* 1887, *1:* 244.

9. Several authors have noticed this sympathy and have explained it as a reflection of Farr's poor childhood. Cullen, *Statistical Movement,* p. 35; and Greenwood, *British Pioneers,* p. 62. Farr was the eldest child of a farm laborer. At the age of eight he was indentured as a parish apprentice, Salop Record Office, Condover Parish Records 1977/7/1882.

10. "Poor law—steam-boiler explosions—coroners' inquests," *Brit. Ann. Med.,* 1837, *1:* 790.

11. "Medical relief of paupers," p. 244.

12. For a brief summary of Farr's disease theory see John M. Eyler, "William Farr on the cholera: The sanitarian's disease theory and the statistician's method," *J. Hist. Med.,* 1973, *28:* 81-87.

13. For further discussion of this tradition see John M. Eyler, "Mortality statistics and Victorian health policy: Program and criticism," *Bull. Hist. Med.,* 1976, *50:* 336-339.

14. "National Board of Health," *Brit. Ann. Med.,* 1837, *1:* 760.

15. William Farr, "Letter to the Registrar-General," *First Annual Report of the Registrar General of Births, Deaths, and Marriages in England,* p. 89 [B.P.P., 1839, XVI, p. 65]. Subsequent references to these reports will be in this form: Farr, "Letter," *1st A. R. R. G.,* p. 89.

16. "Address by W. Farr, M.D., F.R.S. on public health," *Trans. Natl. Assn. Prom. Soc. Sci.* (Manchester, 1866), 70.

17. Farr, "Letter," *Suppl. 35th A.R.R.G.,* p. iv [B.P.P., 1875, XVIII Pt. 2].

18. For suggestions of resentment toward Farr's rhetorical extravagancy see *Lancet,* 1883, *1:* 801.

19. This society should not be confused with the Provincial Medical and Surgical Association which became the present British Medical Association. See Ernest Muirhead Little, *History of the British Medical Association: 1832-1932* (London: British Medical Association, [1932]), pp. 32-34.

20. See for example the following editorials: "Medical competition," *Brit. Ann. Med.,* 1837, *2:* 116; "Curricula," ibid., 430; "Medical reform: Representative bodies v. the corporations," ibid., 563; "Progress of the medical profession—obstructions in the way," ibid., 630; and "The College of Physicians v. Scotch graduates," ibid., 662. Farr's oration was published as William Farr, "Medical reform. An oration delivered at the last anniversary meeting of the British Medical Association," *Lancet.* 1839-40, *1:* 105-111.

21. The best history of this topic is Cullen, *Statistical Movement.* Also useful among other recent works is David Elesh, "The Manchester Statistical Society: A case study of a discontinuity in the history of empirical social research," *J. Hist. Behavl. Sci.,* 1972, *8:* 280-301 and 407-417.

22. The ideals of the statistical movement were well-stated in early published statements by the statistical society of London: "Introduction," *J. Statist. Soc. Lond.,* 1838, *1:* 1-3;

"Sixth annual report of the Council of the Statistical Society of London. Session 1839-40," ibid., 1840, *3:* 1-2.

23. M.J. Cullen has shown rather convincingly how many of the early studies the founders sponsored were biased so as to prove foregone conclusions. The statisticians often "disguised propaganda as facts." Cullen, *Statistical Movement,* p. 144. See also ibid., 106-110 and 135-149.

24. Ibid., 105-115.

25. William Augustus Guy, "On the value of the numerical method as applied to science, but especially to physiology and medicine." *J. Statist. Soc. Lond.,* 1839, *2:* 25-47; Daniel Griffin and William Griffin, *Observations on the Application of Mathematics to the Science of Medicine* (London, 1843); and *Brit. & For. Med. Rev.,* July, 1841, *22:* 1-21.

26. Griffin and Griffin, *Observations on the Application of Mathematics,* pp. 3-8.

27. Ibid., 28-29; and *Brit. & For. Med. Rev.,* July 1841, *22:* 18.

28. Guy, "On the value of the numerical method," pp. 36-38.

29. See in particular *Brit. & For. Med. Rev.,* July 1841, *22:* 16-20.

30. Guy in fact cites the results but not the method Farr used in his study of smallpox to be mentioned shortly. Guy, "On the value of the numerical method," p. 38.

31. *Life Tables, Founded upon the Discovery of a Numerical Law Regulating the Existence of Every Human Being . . .* (London, 1832), p. vi.

32. "On the nature of the function expressive of the law of human mortality and on a new mode of determining the value of life contingencies," *Philos. Trans.,* 1825, *115:* 513-583.

33. The most important of these for Farr's work were: "On the laws of collective vitality," *Lancet,* 1834-35, *2:* 5-8; "On the mortality of the people of England," ibid., 310-316; "On the law of mortality in each county of England," ibid., 1835-36, *1:* 364-371 and 408-416; "On the mortality of infants in England," ibid., 690-694; "On the laws of sickness, according to age, exhibiting a double coincidence between the laws of sickness and the laws of mortality," ibid., 855-858; and "Statistics of the London Hospital, with remarks on the law of sickness," ibid., 1835-36, *2:* 778-783.

34. T.R. Edmonds, "Statistics of mortality in England," *Brit. Med. Almanack,* 1837, pp. 130-137; and [William Farr], "Vital statistics: or, the statistics of health, sickness, diseases, and deaths," in J.R. McCulloch (ed.) *A Statistical account of the British Empire . . .* (London, 1837), *2:* 567-601.

35. Farr's most complete account of his methods of constructing life tables are: "On the construction of life-tables, illustrated by a new life-table of the healthy districts of England," *Philos. Trans.,* 1859, *149:* 839-861; and *English Life Table: Tables of Lifetimes, Annuities, and Premiums . . .* (London, 1864), pp. xiv-xxviii.

36. Edmonds, "On the laws of sickness," and Edmonds, "Statistics of the London Hospital."

37. "On a method of determining the danger and the duration of diseases at every period of their progress. Article I," *Brit. Ann. Med.,* 1837, *1:* 72-79; "On the law of recovery and dying in small-pox. Article II," Ibid., 134-143; and "On prognosis," *Brit. Med. Almanack,* 1838, pp. 199-216.

38. Gilbert Blane, "Observations on the comparative prevalence, mortality, and treatment of different diseases," *Medico-Chirurgical Trans.,* 1813, *4:* 126-130; and F. Bisset Hawkins, *Elements of Vital Statistics* (London, 1829), pp. 4-5.

39. W[illiam] Farr, "A method of determining the effects of systems of treatment in certain diseases," *Brit. Med. J.,* 1862, *2:* 193-195; and ibid., *Lancet,* 1862, *2:* 157-158.

40. Farr, "Letter," *2nd A.R.R.G.,* 95-98 [B.P.P., 1840, XVII, pp. 18-20].

41. William Farr, "Note on the present epidemic of small-pox, and on the necessity of arresting its ravages," *Lancet,* 1840-41, *1:* 352.

42. W|illiam| Farr, "Mr. Lowe and the cattle plague," *Daily News* (London), Feb. 19, 1866, pp. 5-6. For a discussion of Farr's methods see John Brownlee, "Historical note on Farr's theory of the epidemic," *Brit. Med. J.*, 1915, *2*: 250-252; and Major Greenwood, *The Medical Dictator and Other Biographical Studies* (London: Williams & Norgate, 1936), pp. 115-119.

43. |William Farr|, *Report on the Mortality of Cholera in England, 1848-49* (London, 1852), pp. lxi-lxvi. See also Eyler, "William Farr on the cholera."

44. For examples of his earliest attempt see "Diseases of towns and of the open country," *1st A.R.R.G.*, pp. 112-116 |B.P.P., 1839, XVI, pp. 78-80|.

45. Farr, "Letter," *40th A.R.R.G.*, pp. 231-238 |B.P.P., 1878-79, XIX |; or William Farr, "Density or proximity of population: Its advantages and disadvantages," *Trans. Natl. Assn. Prom. Soc. Sci.* (Cheltenham, 1878), pp. 530-535.

46. Edmonds, "Mortality of the people of England," pp. 310-316; and Edmonds, "Law of mortality in each county," pp. 364-371 and 408-416.

47. Edmonds, "Law of mortality in each county," p. 365.

48. See the sections "Diseases of towns and of the open country," in *1st A.R.R.G.*, pp. 108-118 |B.P.P., 1839, XVI, pp. 76-81|; *2nd A.R.R.G.*, pp. 79-88 |B.P.P., 1840, XVII, pp. 9-14|; and *3rd A.R.R.G.*, pp. 98-101 |B.P.P., 1841 Sess. 2, VI, pp. 20-22|.

49. See *5th A.R.R.G.*, pp. 46, 47, 48, 50-51, and 406-435 |B.P.P., 1843, XXI, pp. xxxiii-xxxiv, xxxvi-xxxviii and 200-215|.

50. For a discussion of this controversy and related matters see Eyler, "Mortality statistics," pp. 339-341.

51. Farr, "Letter," *Suppl. 25th A.R.R.G.*, pp. xxvi-xxviii |B.P.P., 1865, XIII|.

Discussion

Alexander Langmuir

Dr. Eyler has made a distinct contribution to the slowly developing literature on William Farr,[1] a titan of the nineteenth-century public health movement, whose importance is only beginning to be appreciated. The short biographical summary by Noel Humphrey,[2] Farr's associate of his later years, remains the best account of his life. But this quite personal and almost current commentary is more an original source than a historical evaluation. Humphrey's greatest service was to extract and organize many of the most relevant selections from Farr's official writings, and make them readily available in a memorial volume published posthumously.[3]

Regrettably Humphrey paid only passing attention to a few of Farr's many contributions to the non-official scientific literature. He was an inveterate attender of national meetings and societies and international scientific conferences. Also he was a close associate of Florence Nightingale and helped her with many of her polemics. Surely Farr's published papers constitute a golden lode deserving deep exploration. The definitive biographer of Farr has discoveries and adventures ahead of him.

Dr. Eyler has explored in depth a little talked about period in Farr's life namely the decade prior to his appointment as Compiler of Abstracts in 1839 in the newly established General Register Office. Farr's first annual letter to the Registrar General,[4] his favorite method of communicating his mature ideas, reveals the depth of his perception of the functions and importance of the office he held. This first letter is one of the great classics of nineteenth-century public health literature and fully supports Eyler's conclusion that Farr had already in the 1830s "coalesced" his basic ideas and "formed the conceptual framework" around which his life time work was to be fashioned.

Eyler's most original contribution at this Conference is the persuasive argument that the actuary Thomas Rowe Edmonds introduced Farr to specific quantitative techniques which were to dominate his career, specifically "the search for a numerical law of an epidemic" and "the use of life tables to measure health and vitality." How important Edmonds' role was vis-a-vis that of Louis and the Parisian School under whose influence Farr came for two years in 1829-31 at the age of 22 I will leave to the Lilienfelds who have delved far more deeply into this period than have I.

I would prefer to talk about other facets of Farr that have become apparent to me as a practicing epidemiologist who was introduced to Farr's contributions by Lowell J. Reed and Margaret Merrell here at The Johns Hopkins School of Hygiene and Public Health as an M.P.H. student in 1939-40. As a lifetime admirer I find it difficult to be objectively critical, but I can try.

Farr's mathematics were fascinating and extraordinary. They were purely functional, even naive but exceptionally penetrating. They expedited some of the most sophisticated contributions to epidemiology of the century. Nowhere in his writings do I find reference to calculus, to Gauss or to the normal curve, or to significance testing. He uses the letter "e" often in his simple algebraic expressions but this is as a constant and not as the base of natural logarithms. He was addicted to exponential equations of simple type but does not refer to Poisson. He uses first, second and even third order proportional differences to construct curves of epidemics without showing any clear perception of the markedly different skewing of the resultant curves he projects.

Brownlee in the early 1900s extols Farr's work on epidemic theory[5] and even promulgates "Farr's Law." Wade Hampton Frost in the 1930s is reported to have stated that Farr's prediction of the subsidence of the cattle plague was "the most courageous epidemiological prediction of all time."[6]

But I find this highly chauvinistic. It seems to me that Farr's Law, so called, can be simply stated that anything that goes up must come down. It always has. Farr was willing without particular reason to take any curve that was convenient. In his study of the cattle plague had he chosen the second difference for which he had two estimates, instead of the third difference for which he had only one, his projection would have been a normal curve, not one skewed to the left, and he would have been right on target instead of foreshortening his predicted epidemic. Farr's studies may indeed have been pioneering and advanced for his time. In effect, they were based on the vague concept of progressive attenuation of virulence with time. This concept has had many recent advocates particularly among microbiologists but has remained unsupported by practical field experience. Farr's epidemic theorizing like that of many others up to the present time did not lead to new fundamental understandings and surely does not warrant the appellation of "Law of Epidemics."

In contrast to Farr's limited mathematical methodologies, Oliver Wendell Holmes, a contemporary American, consulted British mathematicians to perform a highly sophisticated probability significance test on an epidemic of puerperal sepsis.[7]

Nevertheless the impressive feature of Farr's mathematics was its precision and relevance. He regularly used age specific death rates, in fact he often employed the even more precise actuarial rates; he used geometrical rather than arithmetical estimates for intercensal populations, certainly more appropriate in his time; he calculated maternal and infant mortality rates using live births as his denominators. While dealing with many of the most imponderable epidemiological forces such for example as poverty and housing, he always strove for valid comparisons measured with quantitative precision.

Farr was exceptionally well informed about most of the rapidly developing basic and social sciences of his times. His writings bristle with apt quotations from chemistry, economics, history, sociology, demography, and actuarial science. His analogies sometimes seem rather far fetched but always are stimulating. For example in his famous letter about the cattle plague in London in 1864,[8] he describes in detail a comparable epidemic in Rome, 100 years earlier, and reports that the price of beef did not change.

Eyler reports that Farr's "intense emotionally charged rhetoric" was "disquieting" to "his more narrow minded colleagues." Indeed this might be expected. For example, in describing mortality in the influenza epidemic of 1847 where excess mortality was marked not only for deaths ascribed to influenza but also to pneumonia, bronchitis, asthma and many other diseases, Farr states bluntly:

In some of these cases the inflammation specified was the primary disease, in others secondary, and in many it was purely influenza—mis-reported. There is a strong disposition among some English practitioners, not only to localize disease but to see nothing but a local disease.[9]

When cholera returned to London in the late summer of 1853, a year before the great epidemic, Farr showed that mortality in areas served by water from the Lambeth Company which had improved its source, was lower than that in areas served by the Southwark and Vauxhall Company. Although Farr was entranced throughout his life with the relation of elevation above sea level to cholera mortality, he had already accepted Snow's early studies in 1849 on the importance of contaminated water and he wrote in the Weekly Return for December 3, 1853:

It is enacted [by parliament] that it shall not be lawful ["after those dates"] to distribute the pernicious waters over London. It unfortunately happens that in the invasion of cholera with which we are threatened next year (1854), every parish except those which the Lambeth Company supplies, may receive waters as bad as those of 1849 without a direct violation of the Act of Parliament.[10]

He then goes on to emphasize that the improvements could be made "in half the time" due to the "extraordinary emergency."

During the epidemic of cattle plague (rinderpest) that prevailed in England during the fall, winter and spring of 1865-66 a Parliamentary Commission was appointed. One of the Commissioners, a Mr. Lowe, made an alarmist speech in Parliament about the "terrible law of increase" that would bring "a calamity beyond all calculation." Farr wrote a letter to the *Daily News* of London stating:

No one can express a proposition more clearly than Mr. Lowe, but the clearness of the proposition is no evidence of the truth.[11]

These are mere selections of the pithy "emotionally charged rhetoric" which was Farr's almost constant style. There are many definitions of rhetoric and at various ages rhetoric has been in and out of fashion. Alan Gregg's favorite definition was: "Rhetoric is the art of persuasion without resort to reason."[12] Of this I maintain Farr was not guilty. To argue that Farr used emotionally charged language in support of his carefully reasoned and marshalled data there can be no doubt and the epidemiological literature is the richer thereby.

The Farr tradition of the orderly accumulation, collation and publication of mortality data according to a logical system of nosology and along certain highly stylized tabular formats has been maintained certainly in Britain to this day and copied widely through many parts of the world. Unfortunately the practice of writing vividly, and relevantly and fearlessly of the meaning of current statistics did not become a similar tradition.

In a recent visit to the Registrar General's office, now known as the Office of Population, Censuses and Surveys, I was reading about the 1918 pandemic of influenza. Here were the same weekly reports with almost identical tabular arrangement and introductory factual summary statements, describing the tables in the same Farr style. Then the report ends. In mid-October soon after the pandemic had struck in force, there is a slight deviation in the routine text. One line is added: "Beginning with this report a new column will show deaths from influenza." How different would have been Farr's response!

Since 1960 in the U.S.A. and later in many countries an effort to rejuvenate the spirit and tradition of Farr has developed. In that year responsibility for the Morbidity-Mortality Weekly Report was transferred from the Public Health Service, National Office of Vital Statistics, in Washington to the then Communicable Disease Center in Atlanta. Dr. D.A. Henderson, Dr. E. Russell Alexander and I, as a group, endeavored to write meaningful epidemiological commentary to accompany the cold bare statistics. This effort succeeded at least partially.

In 1968 the then Weekly Epidemiological Intelligence Report of the World Health Organization, now the Weekly Epidemiological Record, began to publish current reports of the progress of the Smallpox Eradication Program. Progressively more revelant textual accounts of epidemiological information on a global basis were added. Many countries are now issuing regular surveillance reports in some semblance of the Farr image. The total collective effort has contributed substantially to improved communicable disease control and to wider and prompter communication of current health information to those who have a need to know. The spirit of Farr is reviving.

The time is ripe for a definitive biography of William Farr. I nominate Dr. Eyler.

Notes

1. William Farr, *Vital Statistics: A Memorial Volume of Selections from the Reports and Writings of William Farr*, edited by Noel A. Humphreys (London: Offices of the Sanitary Institute, 1885); reprinted with introduction by M. Susser and A. Adelstein (Metuchen, N.J.: Scarecrow Press, 1975).

2. Farr, *Vital Statistics*, ed. Humphreys, pp. vii-xxiv.

3. Ibid.

4. W. Farr, Letter to Registrar General contained in the *First Annual Report of the Registrar General of Births, Deaths, and Marriages in England* (London, 1839), p. 89.

5. John Brownlee, "Historical note on Farr's theory of the epidemic," *Brit. Med. J.*, Aug. 14, 1915, *ii*: 250.

6. M. Merrell, Personal communication.

7. O. W. Holmes, "On the Contagiousness of Puerperal Fever," 2d ed., with introduction. Reprinted in *Medical Essays* (Boston & New York: Houghton Mifflin, 1891), pp. 103-172.

8. Quoted by Brownlee, "Historical note on Farr's theory of the epidemic."

9. Farr, *Vital Statistics,* ed. Humphreys, p. 332.

10. Ibid., p. 359.

11. Quoted by Brownlee, "Historical note on Farr's theory of the epidemic."

12. Personal communication.

The French Influence
on the Development of Epidemiology

David E. Lilienfeld and Abraham M. Lilienfeld

You may have concluded from Dr. Eyler's excellent review of William Farr's life and times that England was the birthplace of epidemiology.[1] However, it should be noted that Farr spent two years in Paris at a time when medical statistics received a greater emphasis than previously and the French hygienic movement developed. The amalgamation of these two occurrences, as well as the development of mathematical statistics, made France the anvil of epidemiology, where it was first hammered into shape.

These origins will be examined by answering three questions: (1) What actually occurred in France? (2) Why did it occur? and (3) Why did French epidemiology decline in the 1850s at the very time when English and American epidemiology were vigorously growing?

Although Hippocrates has long been acknowledged to be the first epidemiologist, it was not until the appearance of the post-revolutionary Parisian school of medicine that the origin and growth of modern epidemiologic concepts and methods actually began. In the century prior to the French revolution, several developments occurred which had an important influence on the development of epidemiology.

In 1693, Edmond Halley, of comet fame, produced the first known life-table which presented age-specific probabilities of death; this particular life-table was based upon the Breslau Bills of Mortality, sent to Halley by Leibniz.[2] During the next 50 years, such noted mathematicians as Huygens, De Moivre, Fourier, and Bernoulli were involved with the development of the life-table, or as they referred to it, table of mortality. Most of the individuals involved with the early development of the life-table were also astronomers; we propose that this reflected some underlying philosophy that motivated these astronomers to construct them, that is, the discrete mathematical relationships which governed the

28

planets and their movements had biological counterparts, which were known as "laws of mortality." Such relationships were the biological manifestation of more general "laws of nature." For in the seventeenth century, when the concepts of probability and inductive logic were developed, both being essential to epidemiology, the Church-Galilean conflict occurred. Sheynin has suggested that the calculus of probability developed in order to differentiate between natural and divine law.[3] Hence, it is conceivable that these mathematical astronomers' work on life-tables was one way to develop and demonstrate probability concepts, thereby indicating the existence of a natural law rather than a divine one. The development of biostatistics throughout the eighteenth century was premised on the notion of natural laws of mortality. Hence, by the early nineteenth century, a philosophical base for epidemiologic endeavors, that is, elucidating such laws of mortality, had been established. Many of these same astronomers also contributed to developments in mathematical statistics.

The major eighteenth-century political event, the French Revolution, was important for eliminating many previously held medical beliefs and by providing the opportunity for many hitherto neglected students of medicine to contribute their ideas to furthering the healing art. Further, a hygienic movement developed in France.[4] Unfortunately, we do not know all of the details of this movement, but it clearly influenced the development of epidemiology.

Into this environment stepped the eclectic physicians who were to dominate the Parisian school of medicine until the mid-1800s. Some of the leaders of this school can be considered among the fathers of modern epidemiology. The most influential leader in this school was Pierre Charles-Alexandre Louis, who played an important role in the founding of epidemiology. For it was Louis who integrated the philosophical and quantitative concepts that had been developed by the nineteenth century and applied them to the study of disease in order to make inferences on their natural history and etiology, that is, the modern "epidemiologic approach."

That medical statistics were used prior to Louis cannot be denied, for several of his predecessors and colleagues had calculated many "death rates." The theoretical advances in probability and statistics by eighteenth-century French mathematicians, such as Laplace, cannot be underemphasized because they also played an important role. Rosen provides an excellent overview of this development.[5] Nonetheless, before Louis, there had not been a vigorous application of quantitative ideas to medicine.

Many physicians are familiar with Louis' first research project, reported in 1830, on the efficacy of bloodletting. Louis' conclusion, that bloodletting was not very therapeutic, dealt the deathblow to this method. Yet, for epidemiology, this report was important for its description of Louis' conceptual approach to comparative studies, as indicated in this statement:

> In any epidemic, for instance, let us suppose 500 of the sick, *taken indiscriminately,* to be subjected to one kind of treatment, and 500 others, taken in the same manner, to be treated in a different mode; if the mortality is greater among the first, than among the second, must we not conclude that the treatment was less appropriate or less efficacious in the first class, than in the second? . . . that it is impossible to appreciate each case with mathematical exactness, and it is precisely on this account that enumeration becomes necessary; by so doing the errors (which are inevitable) being the same in both groups of patients subjected to different treatment, mutually compensate each other, and they may be disregarded without sensibly affecting the exactness of the results.[6]

Notable is the term "taken indiscriminately"; does this not refer to random sampling? Though this description dealt with the evaluation of treatments, Louis was also quite able to apply these ideas in the field. For example, shortly after his study of bloodletting, Louis was appointed to a commission to investigate the 1828 Gibraltar Yellow Fever epidemic. Time does not permit a presentation of this study, which reflects an unusual degree of conceptual epidemiologic sophistication.

Louis' interests were very broad. Working not only on therapies and epidemics, but also on specific disease entities, he began the differentiation of typhus from typhoid fever; two of Louis' students, Gerhardt and Shattuck, were to complete this work. His study of phthisis is notable for considering methodological issues in such studies and suggesting a method to determine whether phthisis was inherited; Louis stated:

> The tenth part of the subjects who fell under my observation were born of parents, either father or mother, who according to all appearances, had died of phthisis. But, as this disease might have been transmitted in these cases, or have been developed independently of such influence, and as I knew nothing of the manner of death of the brothers and sisters of these patients, it follows in reality that I have observed nothing decisive in favor of the hereditary character of phthisis. I may remark that the proportion of phthisical patients born of parents who died of tuberculosis, is probably below the truth in my notes; inasmuch as it

TABLE 1. Comparison of Annual Rates of Phthisis Among British Troops in Areas with Different Climates*

Area	Total No. of British Troops	Annual Rate of Phthisis per 1,000
Canada	61,066	6.5
Gibraltar	60,269	6.5
Bermudas	11,721	8.8
Malta	40,826	6.1
Home stations in Britain	?	6.4

*P.C.A. Louis, Research on Phthisis, Anatomical, Pathological and Therapeutic, 2d ed., transl. W. H. Walshe (London: Sydenham Society, 1844), p. 492.

is far from being always possible to ascertain from hospital patients the nature of the affection to which their parents fell victim. But it is obvious that in order to substantiate the exact amount of hereditary influence, it would be necessary to draw up tables of mortality, by means of which we should have the power of comparing an equal number of subjects born of parents who were phthisical and who were not so.[7]

It is tempting to speculate that by "the exact amount of hereditary influence," Louis was referring to the attributable risk.

Further, an entire chapter was devoted to the etiology of phthisis.[8] Its organization is very similar to modern epidemiological reports. In attempting to determine the influence of climate and temperature, he presented data on the frequency of phthisis among British troops in areas that differed markedly in climate and temperature (Table 1). He noted that in the Bermudas, with the highest rate, the climate was "mild and equable, while that of Canada is excessively cold, and exposed to great and sudden variations of temperature."[9] He carefully noted that:

No doubt the accuracy of the facts, upon which these statistical results are founded, may to a certain point be made matter of contestation. But errors in diagnosis, which I find no difficulty in admitting must have occurred, did not take place in any single one only of the British colonies; they must have occurred in all, and in about the same proportions; hence the results are strictly comparable. It follows then, from the evidence now brought forward, that the prevailing opinion respecting the influence of climate on the development of phthisis is, if not completely erroneous, at least of most doubtful accuracy,—and that it is either deficient in support of any kind, or rests merely upon the foundation of facts erroneously understood or too few in number.[10]

Although Louis never held a formal appointment in a medical school, he was among the most influential of medical teachers in Paris. In 1834, he published a book entitled *Essay of Clinical Instruction,* in which the practical and philosophical approaches to medicine are presented.[11] In it, he describes how one should take a case history, and some of the methods and problems found in modern observational studies.

> Whether we wish to make a summary of the facts observed during the course of clinical medicine, or to deduce general laws from those collected by the authors, we must, in the first place, assure ourselves of the exactness of the facts; remove from our analyses all of those which are not unimpeachable, and analyze the others *without distinction;* for the object is to arrive at exact results; and by proceeding in the manner pointed out, we make a complete enumeration, and thus take a sure means of avoiding great errors. . . . In order then, that the results obtained . . . should be actually true, it is necessary that the facts on which they are based should be very exact; thus, among the cases where a symptom is wanting, we must not count those where it has not been noted, where no mention has been made of it, whatever may be the exactness of the observation in other respects. . . . But to appreciate the value of a symptom in any disease whatever, we should not only know the proportion of the cases in which it presents itself, but also in what other affections it occurs, and in what proportion, in how many cases it is slight or severe. . . . The numerical method is not less useful in the research of the causes of disease, whether in giving us the means of recognizing serious errors, or in enabling us to avoid them.[12]

Louis was not the only epidemiologically-oriented physician in Paris. Andral appears as another leading one, as well as one of the most prominent hygienists; he was one of the founders of the *Annales d'Hygiène Publique,* the major Parisian preventive medicine periodical. On its editorial board were the leading French hygienists.

Others were also involved in epidemiology during this period: Villermé, for example, analyzed differences in mortality rates by social classes.[13] Also, the renowned statistician, A. Quetelet, was in frequent contact with many in Paris. However, Quetelet's statistical theories were definitely not as "refined" as those of today.

By the mid-nineteenth century, epidemiology in France had declined considerably and its center had shifted to London. One wonders how these ideas were transferred to England. Noting that Louis had attracted many students from England, the United States and Switzerland, we propose that the conceptual basis of epidemiology was transmitted by his students to England and the United States, as shown in Figures 1 and 2. His English students (Figure 1) became the leaders of epidemiology in the middle and latter half of the nineteenth century and included the brightest stars of epidemiology and biostatistics in the preventive medicine constellation.

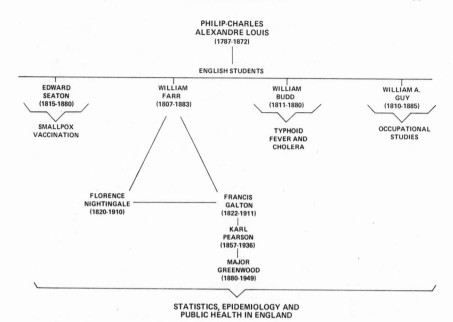

FIGURE 1. The influence of P.C.A. Louis on the development of statistics and epidemiology through some of his students in England.

One such student, William Augustus Guy, forgotten by the medical and statistical worlds, was among the leading biostatisticians of his day. A very active member of the Royal Statistical Society, he served as its president from 1855-1856. In 1854, in one of his epidemiologic studies, he conceptualized what we now know as the odds ratio.[14] William Farr had an astonishing grasp of modern epidemiologic concepts. One interesting accomplishment was his 1837 use of survivorship life-tables, noting:

> The tendency to death or health varies, as the morbid processes themselves vary, every instant from the commencement to the termination of disease. Before examining the intensity . . . of these tendencies, or *forces,* as they are called in physics, it will be well to take a cursory view of the usual succession of phenomena.[15]

The term "intensity . . . of these tendencies" obviously refers to the *force of mortality* usually computed in a life-table. Of course, if the life-table developed as a biological analog to astronomical observations and calculations, this parallel terminology is not unexpected.

Louis' American students taught his ideas in the United States and developed the national vital statistics system so essential to Louis' epidemiologic ideas. These students established two epidemiologic centers in the United States: one in Boston and one in New York. The Boston group included many well-known physicians: George Cheyne Shattuck, Jr., Oliver Wendell Holmes, and Henry I. Bowditch, to name a few. The center in New York resulted from the activities of three of Louis' students; there was Elisha Bartlett, who spent the last five years of his life in New York City, mainly at the Columbia University College of Physicians and Surgeons. Although Bartlett conducted no epidemiologic studies, his understanding of epidemiologic methods was remarkable. Dedicating his *Essay on the Philosophy of Medical Science* to Louis,[16] Bartlett gave examples of both the calculation and use of confidence limits for mortality rates, based on a publication by Jules Gavarett in 1840.[17] Bartlett noted the need for the comparability of study groups:

> The first condition in the establishment of any therapeutical principle or law is this—that the facts or phenomenon, the relationships of which are to be investigated, shall be sufficiently fixed and definite to be comparable. . . . The subjects of the disease, whatever it is, which is to be studied ought to be taken from the same locality and from the same classes of population; and the hygienic circumstances surrounding these subjects, during the treatment of the disease, should be the same. These precautions, it is easy to see, are necessary in order to render the individual cases of the disease *comparable*. . . . There should be no selection of cases. . . . There is one sense in which a knowledge of the normal structure, and the physiological actions of the body may be said to be necessary to a knowledge of its abnormal structure and its pathological actions. We need the former as a *standard of comparison* for the latter.

The latter clearly states a need for a control group.

It is noteworthy that Bartlett was at the College of Physicians and Surgeons at the same time that Elisha Harris and Stephen Smith were students there. They were later to found the American Public Health Association. Also, Harris was the first vital statistics registrar in New York City. The other two students of Louis who taught at the College of Physicians and Surgeons were Francis Delafield and Alonzo Clark. Although not having studied abroad, there was also Austin Flint who had studied at Harvard under Louis' students and upon whom Louis' works had made a considerable impression. Delafield, Flint, and Clark all taught William Henry Welch, interesting him in preventive medicine and epidemiology. Flint was also the teacher of Charles V. Chapin, who became a leading epidemiologist and a pioneer in the public health movement. These relationships are summarized in Figure 2.

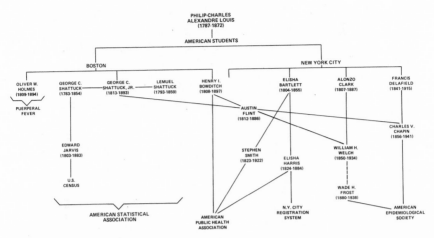

FIGURE 2. The influence of P.C.A. Louis on the development of statistics and epidemiology through some of his students in the United States.

Several parallels exist in the historical development of epidemiology in France, England, and the United States. In France, the underlying philosophy of epidemiology had been developed. Also, the French mathematicians had been active in elucidating various statistical theories, such that, by 1800, a theoretical base for ideas of statistical analysis had been established. Further, an identifiable hygienic movement had developed in France, which was sufficiently significant to warrant comment by British hygienists.

In England, much the same was true. There was an identifiable philosophy of epidemiology, a familiarity with mathematical and actuarial statistics and the development of a well-organized hygienic movement. However, in England, the London Bills of Mortality had been in existence since the late 1500s. Two contradictory reasons have been proposed for their collection: (1) to warn the population of an epidemic so that the populace could leave the city, or, (2) to convince the populace that an epidemic was not so severe for them to leave the city, which would, in turn, disrupt commerce. Several life insurance companies also had been established in England in the eighteenth century and had accumulated a large mass of data concerning their subscribers. Further, the English military had detailed records of troop mortality since the late eighteenth century. Thus, a substantial wealth of statistical data on the morbidity and mortality of various population groups was available in England for analysis. Hence, one difference between England and

TABLE 2. Comparison of Structural Foundations of French, English, and American Schools of Epidemiology

FRENCH	AMERICAN	ENGLISH
HYGIENE MOVEMENT	HYGIENE MOVEMENT	HYGIENE MOVEMENT
STATISTICAL THEORY	STATISTICAL THEORY	STATISTICAL THEORY
UNDERLYING PHILOSOPHY OF EPIDEMIOLOGY	UNDERLYING PHILOSOPHY OF EPIDEMIOLOGY	UNDERLYING PHILOSOPHY OF EPIDEMIOLOGY
	VITAL STATISTICS	VITAL STATISTICS

France was the existence in England of population-based statistics, which we shall refer to as "vital statistics."

In the United States, the situation was similar to that in England, except that vital statistics were not immediately available; rather, vital statistics were developed in the United States by Louis' students. It is apparent then, that the major difference between England, the United States, and France is that the first two countries either had or quickly developed vital statistics, while the last had not. We suggest that epidemiology in France declined because of the absence or non-utilization of a vital statistics system, while epidemiology in England flourished because of its presence and utilization. In the United States, epidemiology developed almost forty years after it had in England; but this period was necessary for the development of vital statistics (Table 2).

Hence, we conclude from this examination of the French impact on epidemiology, that one essential component needed for epidemiology to develop and flourish is the existence, maintenance, and utilization of vital statistics, i.e. population-based statistics; although vital statistics represents only one facet of epidemiology. While previous studies of epidemiology's past history have concentrated on when and what, we believe that it is more important to attempt to determine why and how developments occurred. For, it should be remembered that . . . "Whatever limitations are still obvious, let us not forget that men and methods make epidemiology, not statistical significance levels, nor computers, nor inferences, important as these are."[18]

Notes

1. John Eyler, "The Conceptual origins of William Farr's epidemiology: Numerical methods and social thought in the 1830s," *Times, Places and Persons: Aspects of the History of Epidemiology* (Baltimore: The Johns Hopkins University Press, 1980); see above pp. 1-21.

2. Edmond Halley, "An estimate of the degrees of mortality of mankind, drawn from various tables of the births and funerals in the city of Breslau with an attempt to ascertain the price of annuities upon lives," *Trans. Roy. Soc. London,* 1693, *17:* 596-610.

3. O. B. Sheynin, "D. Bernoulli's work on probability," *RETE,* 1971, *1:* 273-300.

4. Ann La Berge, "Public Health in France and the French Public Health Movement, 1815-1848," Ph.D. dissertation (Ann Arbor, Michigan: University Microfilms, 1974).

5. George Rosen, "Problems in the application of statistical analysis to questions of health: 1700-1880," *Bull. Hist. Med.,* 1955, *29:* 27-45.

6. P. C. A. Louis, *Researches on the Effects of Bloodletting in some Inflammatory Diseases, and on the Influence of Tartarized Antimony and Vesication in Pneumonitis.* Translated by C. G. Putnam (Boston, Hilliard, Gray, 1836), pp. 59-60.

7. P. C. A. Louis, *Researches on Phthisis, Anatomical, Pathological and Therapeutical.* 2nd ed. Translated by Walter Hayle Walshe (London: Sydenham Society, 1844), pp. 483-484.

8. Ibid., pp. 477-508.

9. Ibid., p. 492.

10. Ibid., p. 493.

11. P. C. A. Louis. *An Essay on Clinical Instruction.* Translated by Peter Martin (London: S. Highley, 1834) pp. 20, 23, 24.

12. Ibid., p. 27.

13. Louis René Villermé, "De la mortalité dans les divers quartiers de la ville de Paris, et des causes qui la rendent très différente dans plusieurs d'entre eux, ainsi que dans les divers quartiers de beaucoup de grandes villes," *Ann. d'Hyg. Pub.,* 1830, *3:* 294-341.

14. William Augustus Guy, "Contributions to a knowledge of the influence of employments upon health," *J. Roy. Stat. Soc.,* 1843, *6:* 197-211.

15. William Farr, "On the law of recovery and dying in smallpox, Article II," *Brit. Ann. Med.,* 1837, 1: 134-143.

16. Elisha Bartlett, *An Essay on the Philosophy of Medical Science* (Philadelphia: Lea and Blanchard, 1844), pp. 99, 159-161.

17. Jules Gavarret, *Principes généraux de statistique médicale* (Paris: Beche Jeune et Laube, 1840).

18. David E. Lilienfeld, "The greening of epidemiology: Sanitary physicians and the London Epidemiological Society," *Bull. Hist. Med.,* 1978, *52:* 503-528.

Discussion

Caroline Hannaway

Modern epidemiology is greatly dependent on the use of statistical methods to analyze its data. Looking back in history the development in the nineteenth century of statistical and numerical techniques in the study of population trends, disease incidence, and mortality rates was critical to the rise of modern epidemiology. In their paper, the Lilienfelds have focussed most of their attention on certain aspects of these methodological advances seeking to locate their origin and trace their diffusion in the medical sphere. In my comment I wish to suggest, however, that there was more to the French contribution to the statistical study of disease in this period than the refinement of mathematical techniques and the introduction of concepts used in modern epidemiology—important though these were. We should also ask ourselves what prompted a statistical approach to disease in the first place; what data was thought relevant; and what sort of results or explanations were sought from the analysis of such information. In seeking answers to these questions we may learn much about the historical, medical, and social context in which modern epidemiology arose; and conversely, how a study of the history of epidemiology can both illustrate and illuminate major historical transformations in society.

To illustrate my point I wish to examine trends in French epidemiology over a slightly longer time period than that discussed by the Lilienfelds. I will begin with a discussion of epidemiology in France in the eighteenth century, prior to the Revolution, and then pass on to the period of the post-Napoleonic era dealt with by the previous speakers. The intended effect of this juxtaposition will be to highlight contrasts, although I am aware that transitions could be suggested.

That epidemics were in some primitive sense statistical phenomena was accepted in both these periods. An epidemic continued to be defined as a disease which affected a large number of people with the same

symptoms at the same time. The first attempt in France to give quantitative substance to this definition took place in the last quarter of the
eighteenth century under the agency of a body of which I have made a
special study, the Royal Society of Medicine of Paris.[1] Called into being
specifically to investigate epizootic and epidemic diseases, the Society,
as an instrument of the State, sought to mobilize the governmental
bureaucracy in support of its endeavors. The physicians of the Society
looked to the intendants of the some thirty-four généralités, or districts,
of ancien régime France to transmit to them the relevant data for their
investigation. This use of the intendants was viewed as a natural extension
of their political function: these important provincial figures were not
only the implementors of central administrative policy but had as part of
their responsibility the reporting of significant statistical information
about the population and resources of their districts. In eighteenth-
century terms, the intendants were the political arithmeticians of the
State.

But what data did the physicians deem relevant to their investigations? The controlling element here was the prevailing medical view of
the causative factors in epidemic diseases. In the eighteenth century
these causes were considered to be climatic and environmental, that is
natural phenomena. The notion that atmospheric conditions, the state
of the weather and topography were related to the occurrence of
epidemic diseases, was of course a legacy of the ancient Hippocratic
corpus, but it had been reformulated in the seventeenth century by the
English physician, Thomas Sydenham, in the form of the concept of the
"epidemic constitution." What rendered this concept amenable to attempted quantification in the course of the eighteenth century was the
increased availability of meteorological instruments such as the baro-
meter, thermometer, and hygrometer. As the science of the atmosphere
became quantified so did eighteenth-century epidemiology. Instruments
and charts were dispatched to the provinces to enable tabulation of the
prevailing meteorological conditions and to record the outbreaks of
disease. This was preeminently viewed as a collective endeavor, the
final objective of which was the correlation between climatic (and topo-
graphical) conditions and the incidence of disease. It was believed that if
sufficient data was collected and analyzed some "natural" laws of epidemics would emerge behind the apparent contingencies of the weather
and the ailments of the populace.

The actual computation of such correlations among so many variables was beyond the analytical methods available in the eighteenth

century, even if the principles which stimulated the attempt had been well founded. But what is worth noting in the attempt itself was the effort to locate the causes of disease in nature—it was natural phenomena that were being quantified and analyzed. Dominant in eighteenth-century epidemiology was the notion of man as a product of nature and his natural environment. It is also worth noting the link that was seen between epidemic diseases among humans and epizootic diseases among domesticated animals, for this was part of a program of public health conceived in terms of an agrarian society.

When we turn to the later period around the 1830s in France, we become conscious of different preoccupations. This is the creative period of the French hygienists' movement and contemporaneous with the developments discussed by the Lilienfelds. The new focus is urban; the approach consists of the analysis of the occurrence of disease in delimited locales, instead of being national in scope; and the correlations sought are in terms of social and economic status. The natural and climatic theory of epidemiology has yielded to a theory cast in social terms. The primary quantifiable data for this approach no longer relate to natural phenomena, but to vital statistics, mortality rates and economic data.

A characteristic example of this new outlook is the work of Louis-René Villermé, one of the most prominent figures in the French public health movement, whose activities have been detailed in a valuable dissertation on this subject by Ann La Berge.[2] Villermé's discussion on epidemics with respect to medical statistics and political economy in the *Dictionnaire de Médecine* of 1835 represents, as he says himself, a new way of approaching the subject and does in fact contrast markedly with the more traditional account of such diseases given by Guillaume Ferrus in the first section of the article under the heading of epidemics.[3] Villermé believed that as civilization developed, the frequency and intensity of epidemics had diminished. The poorer classes or those in need were more often attacked by epidemics and, in consequence, were more often victims of them than the wealthier classes. He laid emphasis on the social and economic causes of such disease incidence. In his many studies on conditions in Paris, Villermé based his conclusions on the data collected and organized by Villot, archivist of the Seine district, and Fourier, the noted mathematician and statistician, into the summary known as the *Recherches statistiques de la ville de Paris*. By statistical analysis from such sources, Villermé concluded that poverty and affluence were the main determinants of disease and death. Climate, water supply, location of housing, even population density—the explanations so often previously cited—did not explain the difference in mortality rates between the two groups.

While Villermé and his associates in the public hygiene movement of the 1820s and 30s were highly critical of the inadequacy and lack of methodological sophistication in contemporary French statistics, they made the best use possible of such resources as were available, as their numerous articles in the *Annales d'Hygiène Publique* attest. What characterizes the work of most members of this school, however, is their underlying ideological commitment to the beneficial effects of what they termed civilization in the sphere of public health. The political and economic context of this notion was provided by economic liberalism and the rise of industrialization. This stands in contrast to the physiocratic and agrarian outlook of those who sponsored the investigation of epidemics in the eighteenth century.

This focus on the part of the French hygienists tended to lead them away from the study of epidemics per se into the field of occupational diseases produced by industrial and working conditions. While recognizing the hazards to health of specific working conditions, the majority of the members of this group retained an optimistic outlook on the long-term effects of industrialization and economic growth in providing a better standard of living for all with a consequent reduction in disease.

What I have attempted here is to provide something of the context of the statistical approach to disease in France from the late eighteenth through the early nineteenth century. It is against this background that we must set the methodological innovations noted by the Lilienfelds in their paper. While not wishing to diminish the influence of Louis and his teaching contributions, which arose primarily it should be noted in clinical medicine and were contingent upon developments in that area, to lose sight of the larger picture would be to diminish the French contribution to epidemiology in this period.

Notes

1. Caroline Hannaway, "The Société Royale de Médecine and epidemics in the Ancien Régime," *Bull. Hist. Med.,* 1972, *46:* 257-273.

2. Ann La Berge, "Public Health in France and the French Public Health Movement, 1815-1848," Ph.D. dissertation, University of Tennessee, 1974.

3. "Epidémies sous le rapports de la statistique médicale et de l'économie politique," *Dictionnaire de Médecine,* 2ᵉ ed. (Paris, 1832-46), vol. 12, pp. 145-172.

Epidemiology and the Statistical Movement

Victor L. Hilts

During the cattle plague epidemic of 1866 William Farr wrote what eventually became a famous letter to the *Daily News* predicting that, fears to the contrary, the plague would soon come to an end.[1] This prediction was not based upon any previously established patterns concerning the typical course of rinderpest epidemics, but rested upon a somewhat daring mathematical calculation; noting the gradual slowing of the successive ratios of increase in deaths that had already occurred, Farr extrapolated to the time when the epidemic would peak, and then began to decline. His calculations met with scant respect in the medical community, and the *British Medical Journal* wrote that "Dr. Farr will not find a single historical fact to back his conclusion that in nine or ten months the disease may quietly die out, may run through its natural course."[2] Nevertheless, Farr had the satisfaction of reprinting his letter several weeks later with the observation that the plague had apparently reached its maximum. Eventually the cattle plague did run its course, not exactly as Farr had predicted but nevertheless roughly as hypothesized.

In an excellent "Historical Review of Epidemic Theory" published in 1952, Robert E. Serfling traced the major landmarks in the development of mathematical models in epidemiology and with one exception was able to confine himself to those who did their major work in the twentieth century.[3] The one exception was Farr's letter to the *Daily News*. "Four decades," wrote Serfling, "elapsed between Farr's work of 1866 and the next consequential publication."[4] According to Serfling the next significant publication was that in 1906 by William Hamer.

One cannot fail to be interested in such an historical discontinuity. If Farr's letter of 1866 really had no influence of consequence until after 1900, it would seem that this neglect might afford a case of scientific blindness parallel to that which greeted Mendel's experiments on peas.

43

Indeed, the chronological comparisons are striking, for Mendel also published his experiments in 1866 and they too were only rediscovered at the turn of the century. Questions arise. Perhaps Farr's letter suffered by being published in an unlikely place—the *Daily News*. Perhaps Farr's views could not overcome the resistance of prevailing ideas. Maybe there was difficulty in understanding Farr's mathematical calculations.

Before proceeding with such questions it is well to be sure of the facts. Was there a forty-year hiatus? An attempt will be made to answer this question, and to show that there was no four decade interval between Farr's letter and the next consequential publication in the field of mathematical epidemiology. An attempt will also be made to indicate why the story of such an interval has appeared in the literature. In the process it is hoped that light will be shed upon some problems facing epidemiologists in the interpretation of statistical data during the late nineteenth century.

It would seem improbable a priori that epidemiologists after Farr should have ignored his calculations concerning the rinderpest epidemic. There was a great improvement in epidemiological statistics during the last decades of the century. Not only did epidemiologists after Farr have the constantly accumulating returns from the Registrar General's Office, but as the century progressed they also had an increasing amount of local data as well. English sanitary legislation brought into existence a corps of medical officers of health; and with increasing emphasis on contagious diseases, these officers had as a principal duty insuring that adequate notification took place. By the last decade of the nineteenth century smallpox, cholera, diphtheria, membranous croup, erysipelas, scarlet fever, relapsing fever, typhus, enteric fever, and puerperal fever were notifiable diseases in England.[5] Even earlier several local sanitary districts took a lead in instituting voluntary or compulsory notification of these and other diseases, including measles, whooping cough, and phthisis. The data from the Registrar General's Office made it possible to study statistically the deaths caused by several diseases over a period of years, and local notification made it possible to observe the statistical rise and fall of epidemics in at least some localities on a weekly or monthly basis.

Statistical information thus gathered was often presented in the form of graphs or charts, and these typically revealed a temporal rise and fall of diseases in a more or less random manner but with at least a hint of regularity. Two traditional kinds of analyses could be given to such statistics. First, one could compare localities and attempt to associate observed epidemiological differences with geographical peculiarities. Second, one could examine the data for a given locality and attempt to identify regularities that might be associated with seasonal or meteorological influences. Both approaches were consistent with the sanitarians' traditional emphasis upon environment as the critical epidemiological factor. Had Farr been able to claim in his cattle plague letter that the rinderpest epidemic was dependent upon certain environmental conditions and would subside when these particular conditions disappeared, there would have been no scepticism on the part of the medical community about his predictions. What made Farr's predictions concerning the cattle plague difficult to accept, however, was that the rinderpest was universally regarded as a contagious disease. Why should contagious diseases rise and fall according to definite laws? This was a perplexing question.

It would appear that the first person to be greatly influenced by Farr's cattle plague letter was a Manchester physician, Arthur Ransome (1834-1922).[6] Ransome was born in Manchester at a time when that city, recently beset by the upheavals of the industrial revolution, was a leading center of provincial science.[7] Both Ransome's father and grandfather were Manchester physicians, and his father had been a pupil of John Dalton. Ransome went to Cambridge University, studied medicine at St. George's Hospital, London, and returned to Manchester where he practiced privately and was elected to the chair of public health at Owens College. He also became a leading member of the Manchester and Salford Sanitary Association, an organization which he used to good effect to further his interest in public health and medical statistics. An appointment to the Manchester Hospital for Consumption coincided with Ransome's interest during the latter part of his life in phthisis, a subject on which he wrote many articles. Though primarily known for his writings on preventative medicine, Ransome was also the inventor of the stetometer, a device which led to his being elected a Fellow of the Royal Society in 1855.

In 1909 Ransome said that he still "remembered well" the cattle plague epidemic, Farr's letter to the *Daily News,* and how the "curve followed the course which Farr forecasted in that letter."[8] He also said that "that was one of the first things" which directed his attention to epidemiology. With respect to this last comment Ransome's memory was faulty for he had actually begun his epidemiological researches several years before 1866. In a paper delivered to the Manchester Literary and Philosophical Society in 1860, Ransome investigated the association between several infectious diseases and prevailing atmospheric conditions. He concluded that an increase in temperature is associated with a rise in the incidence curve for measles and a fall in the incidence curve for whooping cough.[9] Nonetheless, Ransome was certainly influenced by Farr's ideas very soon after the cattle plague letter. At the meeting of the British Medical Association in August 1868, Ransome said, "I believe that Dr. Farr, in his letter upon the Cattle Plague, was one of the first to point out the regularity of the course of most epidemic diseses."[10]

Ransome became an avid student of epidemiological statistics, and from the study of these statistics he was soon convinced of the existence of two related phenomena: the "wave of epidemic disease" and the "epidemic cycle." Ransome discussed the wave of epidemic disease in 1868 and may already at that time have begun to suspect the existence of epidemic cycles. Though others had already detected cycles in smallpox and measles, Ransome said that the idea first came to him through a study of his own data on whooping cough.[11] In 1860 Ransome induced medical officers in the Manchester area to notify the Manchester and Salford Sanitary Association on a regular weekly basis of cases of infectious disease in certain poor-law districts, hospitals, workhouses, and other public institutions. As these notifications accumulated, Ransome recognized a biennial periodicity in the whooping cough statistics. Ransome later found what appeared to be similar cycles in a diagram reporting smallpox death rates in Sweden, and with the help of Farr he got in touch with Dr. Berg of Stockholm, then in charge of Swedish death registrations. In November 1875 Berg sent Ransome a list of annual death rates in Sweden indicating the Swedish mortality from scarlet fever, measles, and whooping cough during the past century. Berg's data provided the basis for a chart illustrating epidemic regularities that Ransome used in a lecture on epidemic cycles read before the Manchester Literary and Philosophical Society in January 1880, and in another lecture on the epidemic wave delivered before the Epidemiological Society of London in July 1882.[12]

Being convinced that the waves and cycles detected in his statistics represented true epidemiological laws, Ransome attempted to find the causes involved. There was obvious difficulty in explaining biennial epidemic cycles in terms of annually reacurring meteorological events. Instead, Ransome believed that such cycles could be explained by what might be called a density-of-susceptibles hypothesis; or, in Ransome's words, by the fact that "a certain density of population at susceptible ages is necessary before a disease can spread with the vigour of an epidemic."[13]

> Probably all the facts would be accounted for if we suppose that these disorders can only become epidemic when the proximity between susceptible persons becomes sufficiently close for the infection to pass freely from one to another.
> Exanthematous diseases rarely attack the same individual twice in his lifetime.
> When, therefore, an epidemic has, by either a fatal or nonfatal attack, cleared away nearly all the susceptible persons up to a certain age, then it must necessarily wait a certain number of years before the requisite nearness of susceptible individuals has been again secured.
> There must in the interval be a gradual re-stocking the nation with material fit for the epidemic to feed upon, and it can only spread when the requisite proximity is attained, when the meshes of the network of communication are sufficiently close for it to include all susceptible persons in one grand haul.[14]

Ransome's density-of-susceptibles hypothesis may well have been inspired by Farr's studies relating population density to mortality, but Ransome made no mention of Farr's work along these lines. What Ransome did claim is that this hypothesis would explain the different periodicities of a given disease observed in England and Sweden.

Originally Ransome approached the problem of epidemic waves in the same manner as that of epidemic cycles. In 1868 he suggested that an epidemic spreads through a population of susceptibles in concentric circles like a fire consuming tinder.[15] Given this assumption, he added, it would not be difficult to calculate the curve that would be assumed by an epidemic wave in any district in which the boundaries were known. In fact Ransome had a friend calculate the shape of an epidemic wave in a district with square boundaries, and in 1868 he noted the close correspondence between these calculations and Farr's predictions concerning the cattle plague. Ultimately, however, Ransome chose an entirely different approach for his explanation of epidemic waves.

The history of science is filled with hypotheses that are eminently plausible, but difficult to verify. The hypothesis that Ransome finally adopted as an explanation of the epidemic wave falls into this category. The hypothesis was a very simple one: the rise and fall of the epidemic curve simply mirrors some change in the *materies morbi*. Again Farr had actually led the way. Searching for the reason that epidemics die out, Farr suggested in his cattle plague letter that the epidemic poisons "lose part of the force of infection in every body through which they pass."[16] After 1880 added plausibility was given to Farr's suggestion by Pasteur's discovery of viral attenuation. If the virulence of a virus can be attenuated, perhaps it can also be intensified—and thus account for both the rise and fall of an epidemic wave. With this in mind Ransome published his explanation of epidemic waves in the *Transactions of the Epidemiological Society* in 1882. He wrote, "I am inclined to think that any attempt at an explanation of the epidemic wave should have to rely mainly upon a knowledge of the changes in the degrees of virulence of the epidemic poison."[17]

Ransome never developed his ideas on epidemic waves and cycles beyond where he left them in 1882, but his papers were frequently cited in the epidemiological literature at the end of the century, especially by those who were concerned with measles. Measles was a subject of investigation at this time because sanitary improvements seemed ineffective in preventing outbreaks of the disease, and because bacteriologists—in spite of their noteworthy successes elsewhere—seemed unable to isolate a measles bacterium. Though not always a serious disease, several late nineteenth-century measles epidemics produced significant numbers of fatalities. In 1891, A. Campbell Munro, Medical Officer of Health for Renfrew, adopted Ransome's density-of-susceptibles hypothesis to explain the periodicity of measles outbreaks affecting school attendance at Jarrow.[18] A year later, Arthur Whitelegge (1852-1933), Medical Officer of Health for the West Riding of Yorkshire, argued that a distinction should be made between "minor" epidemics and "major" epidemics of measles.[19] Only the first, he thought could be accounted for "mechanically" as by Ransome's density-of-susceptibles hypothesis; major epidemics, Whitelegge maintained, not only affect more individuals but tend to be more severe and therefore must be associated with a qualitative change in the virus itself. Whitelegge generalized his ideas in 1893 in that year's Milroy Lectures entitled "Changes of Type in Epidemic Diseases."[20] Four years later William Hamer (1862-1936) read a paper before the Epidemiological Society of London in which the various theories of Ransome and Whitelegge were reviewed, and Hamer suggested the importance of considering the age structure of a population in explaining epidemic recurrences.[21] Hamer was an assistant medical officer for the county of London where he worked with Shirley Murphy (1848-1932), who was also interested in epidemic waves and cycles.[22]

In 1906 William Hamer delivered the Milroy Lectures, choosing a title reminiscent of Whitelegge's lectures thirteen years earlier, "Epidemic Disease in England—the Evidence for Variability and Persistancy of Type."[23] Measles, wrote Hamer, is an excellent example of a disease which reveals a persistency of type—the London measles wave has been persistent in spite of "growth of population and alterations of its age constitution, varying customs, and social conditions."[24] A twelfth wrangler in the Cambridge mathematical tripos, the model that Hamer produced to describe this London measles wave was a much more mathematically developed version of Ransome's density-of-susceptibles hypothesis. Whereas Ransome only used this hypothesis to account for epidemic cycles, however, Hamer used it to account for the shape of the epidemic wave as well. Instead of density or proximity, Hamer introduced a "multiplier" that reflected the difficulty (due to geographical or other causes) of an infectious individual coming into contact with a susceptible individual. Where the multiplier could be considered constant (as seemed to be very nearly the case in the London measles wave), Hamer assumed that the number of cases infected by an infectious individual is proportional to the number of susceptible persons in the population. What made these assumptions yield a model was a very clever analysis of the number of susceptibles at several crucial places in the epidemic wave. Hamer noted that at both the peak and trough of the epidemic wave the number of susceptible persons must be the same, since in both situations each case infects one other. Comparing the rates at which susceptible persons were added to the population through birth and were removed from the population by infection, Hamer noted that the minimum number of susceptibles occurs as the epidemic wanes and the maximum number occurs as it rises. Using data from London, Hamer calculated that the epidemic wave, though nearly symmetrical, was in fact skewed.

Without exaggeration Serfling has called Hamer's analysis "a classic model of the epidemic curve of measles and the periodic recurrence of epidemics."[25] It is now clear that Hamer's model was also the culmination of a line of epidemiological thought that ran from Farr through Ransome and included other epidemiologists concerned with the explanation of epidemic "waves" and "cycles." Certainly Farr's letter of 1866 on the cattle plague does not afford an example of scientific neglect comparable to that of Mendel's experiments on peas. We may now return to ask why the story about Farr's neglect should have entered epidemiological historiography. There is a definite answer to this question.

The story about the neglect of Farr's cattle plague letter is directly related to the emergence on the epidemiological scene after 1900 of an entirely new set of statistical tools. It is useful to divide the impact of statistics upon epidemiological thought into three stages. The first stage may be said to have begun with the work of the earliest writers on medical statistics and to have culminated with the work of William Farr. The second stage may be associated with the writings of those individuals who continued the statistical approach to epidemiological topics in the latter part of the nineteenth century but did so with no statistical tools other than those available to Farr himself. The third stage may be said to have begun with the availability in the early twentieth century of new statistical techniques. These techniques did not originate at the hands of the epidemiologists, but were developed by the biometric school, led by Karl Pearson and inspired by the ideas of Francis Galton. The biometricians gave to epidemiology a new mathematical rigor and the language of correlation coefficients, skew curves, and tests for the goodness of fit.[26]

Introduction of the Pearsonian methods did not come easily, and few established epidemiologists did more than learn to calculate a few correlation coefficients. Hamer, for instance, took a dislike to the biometric methods, just as he had previously taken a dislike to the claims of bacteriologists, and in his later epidemiological studies Hamer called for a return to Sydenham's theory of epidemic constitutions.[27] Karl Pearson, on the other hand, had little respect for the statistical techniques already utilized by epidemiologists and called for a new breed of iatro-mathematicians almost as though mathematics had never before been applied to medicine.[28] Among the iatro-mathematicians bred in Pearson's own Biometric Laboratories were Raymond Pearl (1879-1940), Major Greenwood (1880-1936), and H. E. Soper (1865-1930).[29] One epidemiologist who was not a product of the Biometric Laboratories but was nonetheless one of the first to espouse the Pearsonian methods was John Brownlee (1868-1927), the physician-superintendent of the Belvidere Fever Hospital in Glasgow from 1900 until 1914, and subsequently the first director of the statistical department of the Medical Research Council.[30] Brownlee also believed himself to be the rediscoverer of Farr's cattle plague letter.

Having apparently come into contact with the procedures of the biometric school in connection with various statistical questions relating to smallpox vaccination, Brownlee became inspired by Pearson's classification of skew curves and Pearson's method of curve fitting by the method of moments.[31] In a paper delivered before the Royal Philosophical Society of Glasgow in 1904, Brownlee applied Pearsonian techniques to show that the age-incidence curves of several diseases belonged to one of Pearson's family of skew curves.[32] Two years later Brownlee read a much more ambitious paper before the Royal Society of Edinburgh in which he argued that these same techniques would enable epidemiologists to discover the natural laws of epidemics and the causes that determine these laws.[33] Filled with enthusiasm for his ideas, Brownlee opened his paper with the assumption that very little had previously been done to determine the laws governing epidemics:

> The rise and decline of epidemics of infectious diseases have been subjects of interest since the earliest times, but the scientific determination of the laws which govern their course offers even yet a wide and almost unworked field. Not but what a large amount of observation has been made on many of the conditions under which epidemics appear and pass away. Many epidemics are seasonal, and these have been studied; but the lack of any means of determining the course which a given epidemic might have taken in the presence of somewhat different conditions has made the deduction of certain conclusions impossible. Even the laws which regulate solitary outbursts of disease, the special subject of this paper, have been little studied.[34]

In this paper Brownlee argued that outbursts of disease—what Ransome would have called the "wave of epidemic disease"—usually conform to Pearson's skew curves of Type IV.

Brownlee's paper before the Royal Society of Edinburgh was delivered three months after Hamer had presented his model of London measles epidemics, but there is no evidence that Brownlee was familiar with Hamer's ideas.[35] Whereas Hamer assumed a constancy in the infecting organism, Brownlee argued that the shape of the epidemic wave must reflect a "loss in the infecting power on the part of the organism," and suggested that a wave nearly approximating those actually found would result if the infecting power diminished over time.[36] Brownlee seems to have believed that only such a loss in infecting power could explain why the number of susceptibles in the population is never reduced completely to zero—although Hamer's model provided an explanation for this without resorting to change in virulence. While Brownlee ostensibly derived his conclusion that there must be a change in infectivity from an *a posteriori* examination of his statistics, it seems very likely that he was predisposed to such a view on other grounds. Perhaps illustrating this predisposition was a lecture which he delivered before the Philosophical Society of Glasgow in 1908 on the "Germinal Vitality of Nations," in which he similarly argued that the rise and fall of civilizations must be a product of some change in germinal vitality.[37]

Though Brownlee did not mention Hamer in his paper of 1906, he did mention William Farr's cattle plague letter, which he said he had encountered subsequently to his acquaintance with Pearson's probability distributions. Because of his familiarity with Pearson's techniques, Brownlee did notice something about Farr's letter that had apparently escaped earlier writers—that the mathematical calculations used by Farr in predicting the rinderpest epidemic implied that the course of the epidemic would be described by the normal curve of error. Thus Farr's letter appeared to Brownlee as a precursor of the curve fitting techniques in which he himself was interested.[38] In 1915 Brownlee published an historical note on Farr's letter in which he again treated the cattle plague letter as a long forgotten forerunner of the biometric approach to epidemiological law.[39] While recognizing by this time that Arthur Ransome had been acquainted with the ideas expressed in Farr's letter, Brownlee saw no significant developments between Farr and 1900, this assessment was dependent upon his belief that epidemiological laws accounts including that of Serfling.

In conclusion, historians of mathematical epidemiology should not jump too quickly from Farr's work to the twentieth century. Though Brownlee saw no significant developments between Farr and 1900, this assessment was dependent upon his belief that epidemiological laws should be analyzed by Pearsonian methods. In fact, the series of investigations into epidemic waves and cycles that began with Farr's cattle plague letter and culminated in Hamer's model were more important than Brownlee realized. Ironically, it was Hamer's ideas—and not those of Brownlee—that became the basis in the late 1920s for the epidemiological models of H. E. Soper and Wade Hampton Frost.[40] From this perspective there was no forty-year discontinuity in epidemiological thought after Farr, but there was a discontinuity of approach for twenty years after 1906 when the significance of Hamer's results were eclipsed by enthusiasm for Pearsonian methods.

Notes

1. Farr's letter is quoted by John Brownlee, "Historical Note on Farr's Theory of the Epidemic," *British Med. J.*, 1915, *2*: 250-252. For background see Major Greenwood, *Medical Statistics from Graunt to Farr* (Cambridge University Press, 1948), and John M. Eyler, *Victorian Social Medicine: The Ideas and Methods of William Farr* (Baltimore: The Johns Hopkins University Press, 1979).

2. Brownlee, "Historical Note on Farr's Theory of the Epidemic," p. 250.

3. Robert E. Serfling, "Historical review of epidemic theory," *Human Biology,* 1952, *24:* 145-166.

4. Ibid., p. 148.

5. B. Arthur Whitelegge and George Newman, *Hygiene and Public Health,* new rev. ed. (London: Cassell, 1905), p. 451.

6. Obituary notices of Arthur Ransome are in *Brit. Med. J.,* Aug. 12, 1922, *2:* 285-286, and *Lancet,* Aug. 3, 1922, 301-302. A brief notice is in *The Times* (London), Aug. 3, 1922, p. 9. William Brockbank, *The Honorary Medical Staff of the Manchester Royal Infirmary* (Manchester University Press, 1965) contains a notice (pp. 18-19) of Ransome's father, J. A. Ransome.

7. Robert H. Kargon, *Science in Victorian Manchester, Enterprise and Expertise* (Baltimore: The Johns Hopkins University Press, 1977).

8. Arthur Ransome's discussion following papers by John Brownlee, "Certain considerations on the causation and course of epidemics," and Major Greenwood, "The problems of marital infection in pulmonary tuberculosis," *Proc. Royal Soc. Med.,* 1909, *2* (Epidemiological Section), p. 269.

9. Arthur Ransome, "Contributions to medical meteorology," *Proc. Manchester Literary & Philosophical Soc.,* 1860, *1:* 234-236.

10. Arthur Ransome, "On epidemics, studied by means of statistics of disease," *Brit. Med. J.,* 1868, *2:* 386-388.

11. See discussion of periodicities in smallpox (vol. 1, pp. 144-146) and measles (vol. 1, pp. 160-161) in August Hirsch, *Handbook of Geographical and Historical Pathology,* trans. from 2nd German ed. by Charles Creighton (London: The New Sydenham Society, 1883). Hirsch wrote that "there are, in my opinion, two factors only that determine the recurrence of an epidemic of smallpox: on the one hand, the necessary number of persons susceptible of the morbid poison, and, on the other hand, the introduction of the morbid virus." In preparing his entry on "Periodicity in Disease" for Richard Quain's *A Dictionary of Medicine* (London, 1886), J. Netten Radcliffe (1830-1884) had a mathematical friend calculate the interval between two epidemics of equal intensity as follows:

Let p be the number of susceptible people remaining in a population
   after an epidemic.

Let r be the annual excess of births over deaths (all causes), with other
   increments of susceptible population.

Let x be the number of people attacked, or otherwise rendered insusceptible
   during an epidemic.

And let n be the cycle of an epidemic.

To find n

After an epidemic, the susceptible $= p$
Next year   "   " $= p + r$
   "   "   " $= p + 2r$
When the epidemic comes $= p + nr$
After epidemic gone $= p + nr - x$
But this $= p$
$\therefore nr = x$; and $n = x/r$.

12. Arthur Ransome, "On epidemic cycles," *Proc. Manchester Literary & Philosophical Soc.,* 1880, *30:* 75-94; Arthur Ransome, "On the form of the epidemic wave and some of its causes," *Trans. Epidemiological Soc. of London,* n.s., 1883, *1:* 96-107.

13. Ransome, "On epidemic cycles," p. 83.

14. Ibid., pp. 83-84.

15. Ransome, "On epidemics, studied by means of statistics of disease," p. 387 and charts VIII and IX.

16. Brownlee, "Historical note of Farr's Theory of the Epidemic."

17. Ransome, "On the form of the epidemic wave and some of its causes," p. 106.

18. Campbell Munro, "Measles: an epidemiological study," *Trans. Epidemiological Soc. of London,* n.s., 1891, *10:* 94-109.

19. B. Arthur Whitelegge, "Measles epidemics, major and minor," *Trans. Epidemiological Soc. of London,* n.s., 1893, *12:* 37-54.

20. Idem, "The Milroy Lectures on Epidemic Disease in England—Changes of type in epidemic diseases," *Lancet,* Feb. 25, March 4, 11, 18, 1893.

21. William Hamer, "Age incidence in selection with cycles of disease prevalence," *Trans. Epidemiological Soc. of London.* 1897. *16:* 64-77.

22. Major Greenwood, "Sir William Hamer," *Brit. Med. J.,* July 18, 1936, 154-155; M. G., *Lancet,* July 18, 1936, 161. These two obituary notices, written by the same author, are not identical. Obituary notice of Shirley Murphy, *Nature,* May 19, 1923, *111:* 677. Also "Le Docteur Shirley Murphy," *Revue d'hygiène et de Police Sanitaire,* 1902, *24:* 818-823.

23. William Hamer, "The Milroy Lectures on Epidemic Disease in England—The evidence of variability and of persistency of type," Lecture III, *Lancet* March 17, 1906, 733-739.

24. Ibid., pp. 734-735.

25. Serfling, "Historical review of epidemic theory," p. 157.

26. Helen M. Walker, *Studies in the History of Statistical Method* (Baltimore: Williams & Wilkins, 1929).

27. William Hamer, *Epidemiology, Old and New* (New York: Macmillan, 1929).

28. See, for instance, Karl Pearson, "Eugenics and public health," *Questions of the Day and of the Fray,* No. VI (London, 1912). Pearson did not make the task of accepting the new mathematical methods any easier by his linking of biometry and eugenics. Pearson also found himself at odds with the medical community on many specific issues. While the medical community credited the decline in phthisis to improved sanitary conditions and introduction of sanatoria treatment, for instance, Pearson interpreted it as the result of a racial improvement in immunity. In his controversies with the medical community, Pearson was never gentle, as was exemplified by his criticism of anti-typhoid inoculation statistics. See Leonard Colebrook, *Almroth Wright, Provocative Doctor and Thinker* (London: William Heinemann, 1953), pp. 38-40.

29. Lancelot Hogben, "Major Greenwood," *Obituary Notices of the Royal Society of London,* VII, 1950, pp. 139-154. Major Greenwood, "Herbert Edward Soper," *J. Royal Statistical Soc.,* 1931, *94:* 135-141.

30. Obituary notices of John Brownlee are in *Glasgow Med. J.,* 1927, *107:* 290-293; *Lancet,* March 26, 1927, 680; *Nature,* April 16, 1927, 573. "Bibliography of John Brownlee, M.D., D.Sc., F.R.F.P.S., 1867-1927," *Glasgow Med. J.,* 1932, *117:* 203-209. Brownlee's career at the Medical Research Council is mentioned in A. Landsborough Thomson, *Half a Century of Medical Research.* Vol. 1: *Origins and Policy of the Medical Research Council (UK)* (London: Her Majesty's Stationery Office, 1973), pp. 114-115.

31. Brownlee's statistics on smallpox vaccination from Belvidere Hospital were utilized by W. R. Macdonnell, "A further study of smallpox relating to vaccination and smallpox," *Biometrika,* 1903, *ii:* 135-144. Reference to Pearson's journal, *Biometrika,* would have introduced Brownlee to biometric methods.

32. John Brownlee, "Age incidence in zymotic diseases," *Proc. Royal Philosophical Soc. of Glasgow,* 1904, *35,* 301-312. In this paper Brownlee wrote: "The manner in which the mathematical theory of probability is applied . . . is as follows. The form of the curves which represent distributions in the production of which chance is the main factor are first thoroughly investigated. For this Professor Pearson is practically the sole authority. The classes of statistics which it is desired to examine are then tested as to how far they conform with the distributions admitted by the theory. Discrepancy between the facts and the theory, if it exists, can be observed. Of the causes of this, inadequacy in the number of

observations is one. It may also be due, and in the class of fever statistics is commonly due, to the presence of some factor in addition to the most important, namely the age susceptibility, acting specially at some age period [p. 302]."

33. John Brownlee, "Statistical studies in immunity: The theory of an epidemic," *Proc. Royal Soc. of Edinburgh,* 1906, *26:* 484-521.

34. Ibid., p. 484.

35. Robert E. Serfling suggests ("Historical review of epidemic theory," p. 149) that Brownlee "apparently was familiar with the current hypothesis [Hamer, "The Milroy Lectures," 1906] that the progress of an epidemic is regulated by the number of susceptibles, and knew that direct calculation of successive generations of cases, on this hypothesis, led to an epidemic with negative skewness. As he rarely found negative skewness in his observations on epidemics, Brownlee set up a hypothesis that the waxing and waning of an epidemic was primarily the result of a biological change in the 'infectivity' of the organism." There seems no evidence, however, that Brownlee was aware of Hamer's model prior to the writing of his 1906 paper. Brownlee did state ("Statistical studies in immunity," p. 500) that "the assumption that the infectivity of an organism is constant, leads to epidemic forms which have no accordance with the actual facts," but it is not clear that this is a reference to Hamer's hypothesis.

36. Brownlee, "Statistical studies in immunity," pp. 500-502.

37. John Brownlee, "Germinal vitality: A study of the growth of nations as an instance of a hitherto undescribed factor in evolution," *Proc. Royal Philosophical Soc. of Glasgow,* 1908, *39,* 180-204.

38. Brownlee, "Statistical studies in immunity," pp. 484-485.

39. John Brownlee, "Historical note of Farr's theory of the epidemic," *Brit. Med. J.,* August 14, 1915, *2:* 250-252.

40. Serfling, "Historical review of epidemic theory," pp. 149-150, 157-161; H. E. Soper, "The interpretation of periodicity in disease prevalence," *J. Royal Statistical Soc.,* 1929, *92:* 34-73.

Discussion

William G. Cochran

I am glad that Dr. Hilts has given a good deal of attention to the second half of the nineteenth century. My own limited reading in epidemic theory jumped directly from Farr to Hamer, and I knew nothing of the contributions of Ransome and Whitelegge. I don't think, however, that the similar jump in Dr. Serfling's historical review is to be criticized. He was writing a compact review of the historical development of epidemic theory, and naturally concentrated on people like Hamer who actually constructed a theory, working out the mathematical consequences of assumptions about the way in which disease spreads from one person to another.

What struck me from Dr. Hilts' account of the period 1840-1900 was how well the epidemiologists were doing in getting ready for attempts to construct epidemic theories. Through both compulsory and voluntary notification acts, they were collecting regular reports of cases of different kinds of infectious diseases. They were thinking about the nature of any epidemic waves or cycles that they seemed to observe. They were naming and discussing major factors that might explain these features and might be introduced into a theory; in particular, the density of susceptibles in relation to the supply of infectives, changes in the virulence of the infecting organism or in the infectivity of the remaining susceptibles as the epidemic proceeded, the rather vague miasma factor and other meteorological or geographical factors.

This kind of activity impresses me because the period 1850-1900 seems to have been rather quiet and unexciting, with few major breakthroughs, as regards the general development of statistical theory and applications, though I should caution that the period has not been extensively studied. What was happening in statistics? We had Galton's idea of the regression line in 1889, but we had to wait over 30 years until Fisher provided the equipment to put it to full use. The most prolific mathematical statistician of that time, Edgeworth, made some contributions to tests of significance, tests of goodness of fit, asymptotic theory, and estimation, including maximum likelihood. But he created no school, and his name is hardly ever mentioned to students in statistics classes. In the 1890s the heads of Census Bureaus in Western Europe were just beginning to try out sampling methods as a means of saving time and money. The most advanced methodologically of the sampling statisticians was, I think, the Norwegian A.N. Kiaer, who was using and advocating what we now call proportional stratification. The application in which the design of experiments was most advanced at that time was to agricultural field experiments. The agronomists had done limited studies of soil fertility patterns as a guide to the layout of field experiments. The most consistent feature that they found was that adjacent plots tended to give similar yields. Hence, in the layout of comparative trials, the recommendation was that different treatments be placed next to one another. The field of econometrics was further ahead than epidemiology in methods for describing economic waves and cycles, but not, I think, in explanatory theory. My memory may be faulty, but I can recall no work on what I would call causative or explanatory model-building in biology at that time.

The epidemiologists, however, were trying to come to grips with a very complex model-building job. When one thinks of the steps by which infection passes from one person to another with different diseases, it seems clear that construction of a realistic epidemic theory must be a very difficult business indeed. I don't think I was invited here to teach you epidemiology, but let me indicate some of the difficulties in epidemic theory as seen by M.S. Bartlett, the leading mathematical statistician who has worked on epidemic theory. I'll quote in slightly condensed form from his major paper in 1956.[1] He writes:

In spite of the brilliant pioneering work of Farr, Hamer, and Ross, and of important later studies by Soper, Greenwood, McKendrick, E.B. Wilson and others, . . . a quantitative theory of epidemics in any complete sense is still a very long way off. The well-known complexity of most epidemiological phenomena is hardly surprising, for not only does it depend on the interactions between "hosts" and infecting organisms, each individual interaction itself usually a complicated and fluctuating biological process, but it is also. . . . a struggle between opposing populations, the size of which may play a vital role. This last aspect . . . can only be discussed in terms of statistical concepts . . . From the time of Ross at least, the importance of studying the nature, density, and mode of transmission of the infecting agent has been recognized, although reliable information of this kind is often comparatively meagre. . . . The virus or bacterial populations may be in a continuous genetic or other biological state of flux. One need merely recall, for example, the existence of different strains of influenza virus, or the evidence for strains of different virulence in experimental epidemiological studies.

I will add only that the theory must be probabilistic or stochastic, not deterministic. A given set of initial conditions may lead to no epidemic, or to epidemics of different degrees of severity and duration, the outcome depending partly on chance mechanisms. Moreover, because of their mathematical complexity, stochastic processes in time and space began to be tackled relatively late by mathematical statisticians. Proposing conferences is not one of my hobbies—but a case can be made for a short conference of epidemiologists and mathematical statisticians on the future outlook for epidemic theory. The subject offers plenty that is challenging to the mathematical statistician. If the problem of communication can be overcome, the epidemiologists might indicate the kinds of questions of interest to them to which results from theory might help to provide answers.

Given these difficulties, one might wonder why the epidemiologists around 1900 hoped to get anywhere in epidemic theory with the meager tools that they had. Sir William Hamer may have had the right attitude, to judge from his comments on Soper's paper in 1929. He quotes Professor Boycott's advice to take advantage of any specially easy examples that Providence pushes under our noses. He cites measles as such an example, because of the insistent invariability of the measles organism, coupled with the lasting protection afforded by one attack of the disease. He commends Ransome for singling out measles for study, to be followed by Whitelegge, Campbell, Munro and others.

As regards attempts to construct an epidemic theory, Sir William goes on to quote Professor Boycott's warning of the danger of cultivating thoughts and reading books to which we are not equal. But he believed that the Professor would not entirely disapprove of putting our crude ideas about the spread of a disease into some kind of a model, as we would now express it, and seeing how well the model fitted the facts that we know.

Coming to the period after Hamer's 1906 paper, I am not sure whether Dr. Hilts implied that Karl Pearson and Brownlee held up the development of epidemic theory after Hamer. Personally, I doubt whether they or the biometric approach did so. For one thing, I don't think that after 1906 statisticians had the combination of methodology and some knowledge of epidemiology to be able to extend Hamer's approach for quite some time. When I first read Soper's 1929 paper around 1932, I regarded it as a pioneering paper with no obvious fore-runners on the mathematical statistical side.

Soper's paper was very well received when he presented it to the Royal Statistical Society. But the discussants at the meeting indicated the complexity of the problem by noting that the size of the community, the locale—urban or rural—the amount of crowding, and the time of year at which measles start all had an effect on the likely nature of the epidemic. Others noted, as Soper had done, that under-notification and mis-diagnosis made it difficult to check theory against the available data, and still others called for extension of the theory to different diseases, for example, polio.

It is true that Brownlee, as a medical man who was chief statistician of the Medical Research Council after 1914, and as the most prolific writer on epidemics, was in a strong position of influence. However, his insistence that an explanation must fit what was known about the shapes of epidemic curves, now that these could be studied more thoroughly by biometric methods, was reasonable logically. His weaknesses were, I suppose, that he did not think hard enough as an epidemiologist, he did not realize that his biometric data were not very accurate and he was unaware of the complexities of epidemic theory, for which he is hardly to be blamed.

Brownlee did not influence Sir Ronald Ross, who published[2] his mathematical theory of the epidemiology of malaria in 1911 in the second edition of his book. This was a real epidemiologist's theory, based on what Ross knew about the process by which malaria spreads from one person to another. In a 1915 paper[3] Ross was already question-ing Brownlee's pet hypothesis that changes in the virulence of the in-fecting organism were the major factor in explaining the shapes of epidemic curves. In some brilliant work, Ross later developed mathe-matics that extended his theory. This extension could, I believe, take into account both the density of susceptibles and changes in infectivity over time. Ross pointed out that his theory might also be applicable both to other diseases and to crowd phenomena outside of epidemiology.

In conclusion, the layman can find two situations when reading about a period of earlier scientific history. There may be one or two in-vestigators whom I would describe as being just ahead of their time.

They produced fruitful ideas, now taken for granted, that had no visible impact on the development of scientific thought, and were rediscovered years later. On the other hand, as I read Dr. Hilts' account of the period 1840-1900, it seems to show, as he has noted, an orderly and useful progression of ideas.

Notes

1. M. S. Bartlett, "Deterministic and stochastic models for recurrent epidemics," *Proc. Third Berkeley Symp.,* 1956, *4:* 81-109.
2. R. Ross, *The Prevention of Malaria,* 2nd ed. (London: Murray, 1911).
3. R. Ross, "Some a priori pathometric equations," *Brit. Med. J.,* March 27, 1915.

Comment

Owsei Temkin

Though several speakers may have alluded to it, it should be stated clearly that epidemiology as discussed rests on the distinction of separate diseases, or clinical entities. As long as all epidemics of severe illness were comprised under the term "plague," the individual illnesses could not be evaluated statistically, and they had no individual history. The separation of epidemic illnesses into the forms now known proceeded but slowly; it is only necessary to remember how late diphtheria was definitely recognized as a specific disease and typhus and typhoid distinguished from one another. In the forties of the nineteenth century this process met with opposition from the so-called physiological school that was particularly strong in Germany (Wunderlich, the young Virchow, Traube)[1] but was also represented elsewhere, e.g. by Hughlings Jackson in England.[2] Only the rise of bacteriology reestablished a firm belief in specific diseases. Where disease entities are thought of as conceptual artifacts of no more than practical value they are likely to be denied historical existence. It would, therefore, be interesting to investigate the attitude of the physiological school toward epidemiology and the role it played in its development.

Notes

1. Knud Faber, *Nosography: The Evolution of Clinical Medicine in Modern Times,* 2nd ed. (New York: Hoeber, 1930), ch. 3, pp. 59-94.
2. Cf. Owsei Temkin, *The Falling Sickness,* 2nd ed. (Baltimore: The Johns Hopkins University Press, 1971), p. 339.

Attempts at the Eradication of Pellagra: A Historical Review

Daphne A. Roe

The disease pellagra has traditionally been associated with the consumption of a diet with maize as the staple cereal. The first observations of pellagra were made in 1735 by the Spanish physician, Gaspar Casal, who found it was a common cause of ill health and early death among the peasants of the Asturias. His description of the disease, then termed "mal de la rosa," was published posthumously in 1762.[1] Casal recognized that "mal de la rosa" was a multi-system disease which affected the poorest laborers in the Asturias, who lived on a maize diet, varied only by the addition of turnips, chestnuts, cabbage, and occasionally beans, nuts and apples. The common food of the Asturian laborers was an unleavened corn bread made by mixing corn meal and water and baking the mixture in the cinders. Although Casal considered "mal de la rosa" a disease associated with peculiar climatic conditions of the Asturias, he also realized that it was a disease induced by an inadequate diet, and that it could be effectively treated by changing the diet so that milk, cheese and other protein foods were made available to the indigent in the local population.

By 1740, pellagra was recognized in northern Italy and thereafter, it spread rapidly so that in 1784 Gaetano Strambio, who wrote extensively on this subject, calculated that about one-twentieth of the population of Lombardy had pellagra.[2] In the districts that were most affected by the disease, he estimated that there was one pellagrin among every five or six individuals. After the middle of the eighteenth century, the geographical distribution of endemic pellagra and its spread followed the adoption of a corn diet as a means of feeding laborers in countries where sharecropping was practiced.[3]

While there is evidence that pellagra may have existed as a sporadic disease prior to the introduction of maize as a commercial crop, it can be stated that at least in Europe and later in Egypt, South Africa and the United States, pellagra as an endemic disease did not occur until at least 50 years after the establishment of a maize economy. For example, in France, maize was first grown extensively in the latter part of the eighteenth century. In 1790, Arthur Young, the agriculturalist, traced an oblique line across the map of France to divide the northern areas where corn would not ripen from the southern areas where corn was easily produced. In 1829, the French Horticultural Society sought to encourage the development of the corn crop in the environs of Paris. Louis Phillipe, then the Duke of Orléans, planted a tremendous acreage of maize in his land at Neuilly and was given a medal by the Society for his example, but that same year pellagra was reported in the Landes in southwestern France.[4]

Pellagra — The Disease

Pellagrins, or those who have pellagra, characteristically suffer a protracted illness. Physicians have usually divided the course of the disease into four stages. The first is marked by vague symptoms, including headache, malaise, neck pains, dizziness, weakness, particularly in the legs, and hypersensitivity to touch. In the second stage the skin becomes sensitive to sunlight and exposure to the sun causes the development of a chronic dermatitis of the exposed portions of the skin. Occasionally, the skin lesions may develop after other forms of injury such as exposure to excessive heat from stoves. Soreness of the tongue and mouth, accompanied by great thirst, may develop in the disease or may be coincidental with the second stage. The third stage is characterized by the appearance of severe disturbances of the central nervous system. The patient experiences abnormal burning sensations of the hands, abdomen, shoulders, arms, and feet, and suffers from an almost constant headache. However, the most prominent symptoms are of mental illness with profound psychotic depression. Delusions of persecution or sin are not uncommon. Some pellagrins show suicidal tendencies. Refusal to eat is a serious complication and in a debilitated patient can lead to starvation. The last stage is one of wasting with increasing weight loss, diminishing strength, and a tendency to succumb to intercurrent disease such as tuberculosis or other infections.

In a northern temperature climate, the first symptoms usually develop early in the year. The second stage appears as the season advances and there is more sunlight. These symptoms, particularly the
dermatitis from light exposure, last about three or four months, during
which time the skin becomes pigmented over the affected parts. Then
the condition tends to recede and the pellagrin may appear to recover.
During succeeding springs, however, the disease will reappear with
increasing severity so that the patient may pass gradually into the later
phases. Wherever endemic pellagra has occurred, the mortality has
been related to prolonged nutritional deprivation.

Whereas we have known since 1937[5] that pellagra is due to a deficiency of the B vitamin, niacin (nicotinic acid), there is much evidence
to support the thesis that in endemic pellagra other nutrient deficiencies
may also be present, including protein deficiency and deficiency of
another B vitamin, namely riboflavin. Multiple nutritional deficiencies
in pellagrins are readily explained, both by the nature of their diet and
also by the fact that niacin deficiency itself causes changes in the small
intestine which impair the absorption of other nutrients. While the
common dietary staple of populations with endemic pellagra has usually
been corn, the disease has also occurred in people living on millet.
However, the most uniform feature of the food supply of people who
have developed pellagra has been a gross lack of protein foods including
milk, cheese, meat, fish, and eggs. These protein foods are sources of
niacin and of the essential amino acid, tryptophan, which is an en-
dogeneous source of niacin.

Theories of Pellagra Causation

Formal development of theories to explain the occurrence, development and spread of pellagra date back to the latter years of the eighteenth
century. It was at this time that the idea that corn was the sole cause of
pellagra was first proposed. Francesco-Luigi Fanzago emphasized the
association of corn consumption and pellagra as early as 1789, and in
1807 he read a report before the Academy of Medicine in Padua, in
which he stated that maize was the cause of the disease.[6] Three years
later, another Italian pellagrologist, Giovanni Battista Marzari, set forth
his ideas on the causation of pellagra which were to be elaborated by the
proponents of the so-called "Zeist theory" (the belief that pellagra is

caused by a maize diet). He believed that a corn diet could cause pellagra for two reasons: firstly, because the corn, as consumed by the Italian peasants, might be moldy, and secondly, because this cereal was low in nitrogenous material. His observations on the ill effect of a corn diet may be summarized in a translation in his own words:

The appearance of the disease is preceded by the continual use of a vegetable diet throughout the winter season. This diet is composed of Turkish wheat which is almost entirely of the cinquantino type, never quite ripe, sometimes moldy which in our locality is made into polenta often without even salt for seasoning. This monotonous food forms at least 95% of the total diet of the peasants throughout the winter and in the spring; they may have an addition of a few vegetables such as cabbage cooked in water or skimmed milk, but practically never any eggs because they are too expensive. They may have lettuce or chicory which grows wild. . . . The alderman and the Carmelite nuns eat fish and "fast" constantly, but they never get pellagra like the field laborer; their rations are 20 times more ample than those of the peasants and they live on them without any health problem. . . . It must be seen besides that during the long and cold seasons of winter, field laborers, living on this debilitating regime lead an idle, miserable life lying down for many hours of the day and during the long nights in the stables with the animals, thinking of their debts and of what will become of their jobs and of the necessities of each day and of the impossibility of meeting their commitment, and particularly of their complaints against all men who disturb, menace and oppress them. I have many times observed that if a villager passes rapidly from a state of comfort to one of misery, then this is soon followed by a crisis, a cachexia or period of withering away in which the pellagrin, in addition to his other ills, fails in the last degree and comes to a sad end. You will find that two things constantly precede the appearance of pellagra: the first is the continual use of corn or Turkish wheat, where the diet is only a vegetable source; the second is the idleness of winter . . . which is the time of growth of the germ of this disease which is regularly developed by the light or the heat of the springtime.[7]

This description suggests that Marzari was familiar with the complex etiology of the disease, including such factors as the exclusively cereal diet of the pellagrin, particularly during the winter, which put the peasant at nutritional risk; the exposure to sunlight in the spring and summer which caused development of the skin signs of the disease; and perhaps much more importantly two other factors, namely, the economic distress of the peasants and the fact that they were condemned to live on a subsistence regime which was virtually devoid of animal protein.

Harriet Chick, the British nutritionist, pointed out that since there was no knowledge of the nutritive values of specific foods before the end of the nineteenth century, earlier scientists could only guess at reasons why maize should be less nutritious than wheat or other cereal and somehow causative of pellagra.[8]

In order to explain the ill effects of corn consumption as a staple, theories were developed suggesting that maize, particularly moldy maize, contained a toxic material. While some investigators believed that the toxin might originally be present in the grain, most of them thought that the toxin was developed after the harvest, when the maize was stored under damp conditions, so that it became infested with molds or fungi. As time went on, Zeist doctrine became more and more complex and often quite divorced from reality. Blind adherents to Zeist theory would not countenance proposals for the prevention or cure of pellagra by methods which were not based on their beliefs. The most famous exponent of the Zeist theory was Cesare Lombroso, who was born in 1836 at Verona. He studied in Padua, Vienna and Paris, and in 1862 became professor of psychiatry at Pavia, later director of the Insane Asylum at Pesaro, and then holder of the chair of Criminal Anthropology at Turin. His chief scientific interests centered on the relationships between mental and physicial disorders, and his principal claim to fame was his contention that criminals could be identified by certain physical characteristics. However, he spent about 25 of the latter years of his life almost exclusively in the study of pellagra. His belief that pellagra was caused by the eating of spoiled corn came to be known as Lombroso's theory. Lombroso's final conclusion was that pellagra was an intoxication produced by the action of certain organisms on maize. These organisms were considered to be harmless in themselves, but it was believed by him that they possessed the property of producing a poisonous ptomaine when they came in contact with the kernel of the maize. The particular microorganism which was incriminated was Sporisorium maidis.[9] Lombroso's influence on pellagra theory continued until the twentieth century as evidenced by W. C. Sullivan in 1901:

Pellagra, as Lombroso has shown, is dependent on intoxication by diseased maize. Increased dearness of corn (wheat) necessarily leads to its replacement by maize in food of the people; and the price of maize rising with the increased demand, inferior and diseased quantities are consumed, and pellagra becomes more prevalent. The corn (wheat) tax in Italy, which keeps the price of the grain at 25 lire per quintal as compared with 14 lire in London and New York, thus operates as a powerful agent in the increase of pellagra.[10]

Zeist theory was not always a barrier to progress because some of the believers could debate the rigidity of the doctrine and by broadening their theoretical base for the causation of pellagra did contribute to the control of the disease. Thus, Théophile Roussel, who was a determined proponent of the Zeist theory, succeeded in introducing agricultural reforms which led to the conquest of pellagra in France. He put forward the hypothesis that pellagra was the result of both extrinsic and intrinsic factors. According to Roussel, a diet of damaged or rotten corn would cause pellagra only in poor people whose heredity gave them a peculiar susceptibility to the disease.[11] Like Marzari, he also believed that pellagra only developed in people who could not obtain a diet with an adequate supply of foods of animal origin.

Anti-Zeist theories were perhaps equally detrimental to progress in the conquest of the disease. Pierre Thouvenel believed that pellagra was caused by bad air.[12] He explained the extensive occurrence of pellagra in northern Italy by pointing to the extension of irrigation canals in the Lombardy plain by which large amounts of stagnant water were produced with a constant mist covering the whole area. This, he thought, led to a "dephlogistication" of the atmosphere and when debilitated peasants breathed this air they contracted pellagra. Although Thouvenel believed that the excessive humidity played an important role in the cause of pellagra, he also thought that the diet of the pellagrin might play a subsidiary role. Thouvenel may have been influenced by Casal's original meteorological observations of the area in northern Spain where endemic pellagra first occurred, but it seems more likely that his theory was largely based on traditional ideas about the causes of epidemic disease.

Another theory which obtained considerable support in Italy was the idea that the disease was caused by "insolation," or an excessive exposure to sunlight. This idea originated in a monograph by Frapolli (1771), in which pellagra was attributed to the sun's rays and a belief established that the disease was, in fact, a variant of sunstroke.[13]

In France in the mid-nineteenth century, pellagra was first seriously thought of as a disease of the indigent who lived in unsanitary, over-crowded conditions. The pellagra syndrome was spoken of as the "morbus miseriae." Pellagra as a disease of those who lived under wretched circumstances, stemmed from observations in the Landes where the disease was largely confined to people living in hovels in marshy areas. Jean Hameau, who first described pellagra in this area, and more particularly his son, J.-M. G. Hameau, while noting the association of pellagra with poverty situations, thought the disease due to an infec-tion.[14] Hameau, the younger, thought that pellagra was transmitted from sheep to human beings when peasants lived in the same hovels as their animals. However, those who supported the idea that pellagra was a contagion also insisted that vulnerability to the infection was due to the co-existence of "bad blood." As late as 1916, Charles Davenport, a famous American geneticist, wrote: "It appears that certain races or blood lines react in the pellagrin families in a specific and differential fashion that will go far to prove the presence of a hereditary factor in pellagra." He believed that pellagra was communicable and that the progress of the germ in the body depended on constitutional factors.[15] When we consider these rather fantastic ideas, we must remember that it was frequently observed that pellagrins were likely to occur in groups and in families, and the assumption was made, therefore, that these people had in common "bad blood" and/or that they caught the infection from one another.

With the development of microbiology in the latter years of the nineteenth century and the early twentieth century, it was shown that many infectious diseases had an insect vector. The idea that pellagra was due to an infection gained further support. For example, Louis Sambon, a British physician and biologist, noted for his work on the role of the tsetse fly and trypanosomiasis, believed that pellagra was an insect-borne disease carried by a blood-sucking fly of the genus *Simulium*.[16]

Pellagra Eradication

Early in his medical career, Roussel noted relationships between dietary inadequacy and pellagra. In 1845, he described his conviction that both the medical profession and the government in France should recognize the need to augment the quality and quantity of food available to poor people living in endemic pellagra areas. He particularly urged provision of more food derived from animal sources. In stating his viewpoint, which he had developed as a result of studies of pellagrous communities, Roussel, in his *Traité de la pellagre et des pseudo-pellagres* (1866), explains his position as follows: "I admit that you can't argue the point which is agreed by economists of our day that people of the class which provides pellagrins owe a part of their inferior physique and morale to their suffering and to their insufficient food and to their excessive use of a vegetable diet."[17]

He refers to statistics obtained by Longchamp showing that up until 1840 meat consumption in France was about 20 kg. per capita per year, whereas in England at the same period meat consumption was about 82 kg. per capita per year. Roussel pointed out that the 20 kg. figure for meat consumption in France was further misleading because it was an average which overlooked the fact that actual meat consumption of the people in pellagrous communities was limited to salt pork or fatback.

Despite his recognition of the fact that pellagrins ate a diet lacking in animal protein, Roussel's 1845 proposals for the prevention of endemic pellagra were almost entirely a reflection of his Zeist philosophy. He advised research on varieties of maize, adapted to the climate and growing conditions of the areas where pellagra occurred. In France, this area was the southwest, including the Landes and the Pyrénées. Based on the experience of Italian physicians, and the advice of French agriculturalists, he suggested that strains of maize known under the names "quarantain" and "cinquantain" should not be grown for food because they were subject to blight. Secondly, he advised that methods be devised for the efficient oven-drying of maize to prevent mold growth and conservation of maize after milling to preserve flour in the dry condition. Thirdly, he emphasized a need, in using maize flour to make bread, of combining it with wheat flour (one part corn to two parts wheat flour) so as to increase the gluten content and the nutritional value of the product. Alternatively, he suggested that the corn should be used to make a *gaude* by mixing the maize flour with milk as well as water. In 1848, he wrote to the French Minister of Agriculture and described findings of his field studies with the French Pellagra Commission during 1844. At this time he had made an extensive tour of southwestern France and had investigated the food habits and social conditions in pellagrous communities. In the letter to the Minister, he justified the viewpoint that the affected peasants' food must be changed. Realizing that extreme poverty conditioned the eating habits of these people, he was pessimistic about any immediate social progress and about legislation which might ameliorate the lot of the French peasants in areas such as the Landes, where distribution was based on the product of a sharecropping system and barren land. According to Roussel, an improved way of life for the peasants could only come gradually and this was not the responsibility of physicians such as himself. Rather he thought that endemic pellagra could be wiped out by implementing recommendations for change in maize culture processing and preparation. Roussel's recommendations were largely adopted and the conquest of pellagra in France followed, though not altogether as a direct result of his advice or of the application of his policies.

Bordier, writing in 1884,[18] mentions that by that time pellagra was rarely seen in French towns of the endemic areas because although the inhabitants still ate polenta, they ate other food as well. He goes on to

assert that in the Landes the incidence of pellagra had diminished because the maize was dried in ovens, and he further mentioned that the
quarantain and other mold-susceptible strains of maize had been replaced
by other varieties named ellitico, aurao and pulilis; and finally he considered the success of pellagra eradication to have resulted from medical
treatment with arsenic!

We know that, in addition to the implementation of Roussel's three-
point recommendations, it became the French government's policy to
encourage animal husbandry in the Landes and promote cultivation of
cereal crops other than maize. The disease persisted in small areas of
southwestern France until the beginning of the twentieth century. The
pockets of residual endemic pellagra can perhaps be explained by continued poverty and ingrained food habits which limited the peasant's
diet. Pellagra was not entirely wiped out in France until the economic
conditions in the Landes and surrounding areas were drastically improved in the first decade of the twentieth century. Marie in 1908
described the remarkable changes that had occurred:

They made of a marshy waste a rich and fertile country by the exploitation of
seacost pines and by the cultivation of better cereals even of the vine, all accom-
plished by the marvelous works of drainage, which are the glory of the government of that region. . . . Corn is still cultivated, and is even still eaten; but it is in
part given to stock; and even if it is used for human food, there is added wheat
or other cereals, legumes, and also meat and wine. . . . Today the Landes has
railroads, which guarantee the transportation of foodstuffs of all sorts. Intelligence, the will of individuals, the aid of the local government, such are, if not
the entire prophylaxis against pellagra, at least the instruments of this great
work.[19]

Looking back, we can see that the conquest of pellagra in France
was, in fact, triggered by Roussel's concern for the problem of the
quality of the French peasants' diet. Thus, although his ideas for the
prevention of the disease were based on an unproven theory, that is on
the idea that pellagra is caused by the eating of moldy corn, he nevertheless brought the seriousness of the matter to the notice of the French
government, and spurred the government on to take what proved to be
appropriate action.

Pellagra as a Protein Deficiency

Let us now turn to a totally different approach to pellagra prevention
and cure, based on the assumption that the disease is caused by a dietary

deficiency. By the time of World War I, the concept of deficiency diseases was well developed. Indeed, in 1913, Sandwith suggested that the reason maize eaters developed pellagra was because the protein, zein, present in the corn, was deficient in tryptophan. In the following year, Lorenz demonstrated that high protein diets were curative in pellagra.[20]

At the same time, Joseph Goldberger, of the U.S. Public Health Service, was appointed by the then Surgeon General, Rupert Blue, to evaluate the pellagra problem which by then had reached epidemic proportions in the southern states. In his first investigation of pellagra in southern institutions, Goldberger observed a peculiar immunity of the nursing staff and institution attendants to the disease. He then found out that such staff had the privilege of selecting the best food and had access to outside food supplies which they could purchase when off duty. Starting with this information, he and his colleagues studied the diet of children in orphanages where pellagra was a recurrent problem. Through these investigations, Goldberger became convinced that cereals and vegetables formed a much greater proportion of the total food intake of children in these institutions than of the food of well-to-do people who, as a class, were practically exempt from pellagra. Goldberger lost no time in putting his ideas to practical tests. He decided to find out if, by altering the diet of the children in two selected orphanages in Jackson, Mississippi, he could prevent pellagra occurrence among the children. The milk supply was increased so that each child under 12 had 7 ounces of milk twice daily; those under 3 had milk three times a day. Buttermilk was also supplied for children, and they received an egg a day, and beans and peas at the midday meal. The breakfast cereal was changed from grits to oatmeal, and meat, instead of being served once a week, was served three to four times a week. After one year, only one case of pellagra occurred within these two institutions.[21]

Goldberger's modest and local success in pellagra control, as well as his subsequent induction of pellagra in prison inmates by feeding them a diet similar to that of the pellagrins was rapidly published and soon came to the attention of William H. Wilson, professor of physiology in the School of Medicine in Cairo. Wilson not only knew about the history of pellagra, but he also had familiarity with current knowledge of protein requirements. In 1919, due to the frequency of pellagra recurrences in the Abbassia Asylum for the Insane in Cairo, he was asked to report on whether the diet of the institution, which appeared to be adequate for normal persons, was in any way defective. In his report on the diet of this asylum, he commented:

The rations, in addition to other articles, contained 100 g. of meat, 50 g. of milk, and 300 g. of fresh vegetables. The calorie value was sufficient. It was thought however that as the minimum protein requirement of a pellagrous and insane community was likely to be higher, possibly considerably higher, than the normal [regarded by Wilson as equivalent to 40 g. of animal protein] it would be well to increase the protein. This was done by the addition of 45 g. of meat and 50 g. of milk. . . . During the following year the death rate from pellagra in this institution was diminished by nearly 50%.[22]

This experience, coupled with Wilson's knowledge of etiological factors known to influence the occurrence of endemic pallagra, led him to the following conclusions:

1. The chief etiological factor in pellagra is a deficiency of protein in the food and this is best determined by an estimate of the biological value of the protein.

2. Large individual variations occur in the minimum requirements for protein but the lower the biological value of the food protein, that is, the lower the amount of nitrogen from that protein that is retained by the body, the larger the proportion of persons who develop pellagra.

3. The level of protein requirement is raised by labor if the energy intake is deficient, by a previous attack of pellagra and by illness, especially chronic disease of the alimentary tract.

Further, based on the scientific work of Karl Thomas, he was able to estimate the biological value of specific food proteins. Careful analysis of the diets of pellagrins led him to the conclusion that the disease was brought about by the habitual consumption of corn in which the protein, zein, had a low biological value. Acceptance of this theory produced the further hypothesis that prevention as well as cure of the disease would result from addition of proteins of high biological value to the diet of people having the disease or at nutritional risk. He also recognized that, in general, pellagrins consumed very little total protein and yet their requirements were very high. These logical conclusions, despite certain flaws which have since been determined, were applied to eradicate pellagra in an Armenian refugee camp at Port Said. The camp was a few miles from Port Said and was located in the desert of the Syrian side of the Suez Canal. About 3,840 refugees, coming from northern Syria and southern Asia Minor, where they had endured great physical hardships, were received by the British and brought to Port Said in September 1915; organization for their relief was established and food was supplied to the camp. In 1916, pellagra was discovered among the refugees, and about 10% of the camp population was affected. Dr. R. G. White, of the

TABLE 1. Distribution of Armenian Refugee Camp Population by Age and Sex

Age	Males	Females	Both Sexes
0-4	265	253	518
5-14	470	480	950
15-20	371 ⎫	372 ⎫	743
21-30	199 ⎬ 1022	338 ⎬ 1350	537
31-40	137 ⎭	236 ⎭	373
41 & over	315	404	719
Total	1757	2083	3840

Based on W. Wilson (n. 20), p. 17.

TABLE 2. Percent of Cases of Pellagra in Armenian Refugee Camp by Age and Sex

Sex and Age group	Number in Population Group	Pellagra Cases No.	% of Population
Males			
0-14	735	54	7.4
15-50	812	34	4.2
Females			
0-14	783	66	8.4
15-50	1071	329	30.7

Based on W. Wilson (n. 20), p. 19.

Egyptian Public Health Department, was sent to investigate, and he reported on the demographic characteristics of the camp population. His statistics are shown in Tables 1 and 2. Commenting on the preponderance of females over males who had pellagra, Wilson suggested that the women were at particular nutritional risk because it was an ingrained habit of Armenian women to share their food with their husbands and children. This custom, together with the already restrictive food supply and hard work required of the women in nursing a sick household, were believed by Wilson to be contributory factors which, together, would explain the high incidence of the disease in camp women.

In collaboration with Dr. White, Wilson changed the camp diet. The first change to be made was the addition of lentils and beans but, unfortunately, due to food prejudices among the camp population, this leguminous diet was not well received and after two months, that is in February 1917, two further diets were provided to the camp residents. One of these diets was for adults who had not suffered from pellagra, and the other was introduced specifically as an anti-pellagrous diet, and was given to all persons who had suffered from pellagra in the previous

TABLE 3. Original Deficient Diet of Armenian Refugees in Port Said Camp, 1916.

Article of Diet	Daily Amount in gm.	Gross Protein	Available Protein	Biological Value of Protein
Bread	750	—	37.5	15
Bourghoul	5.5	—	.5	.2
Cheese	17.1	—	2	2
Meat	8.6	—	1.6	1.6
Oil	5.3	—	—	—
Lentils	11	—	2.1	1.17
Beans	7.1	—	1.3	.7
Rice	8.6	—	.56	.5
Sugar	18.8	—	—	—
Vegetables	53.4	—	.53	.25
Onions	2.5	—	.03	.01
Olives	14.3	—	.11	.05
		57	46.2	21.4
Value of diet for adults (over 14 years)		64	51.5	23.0

Calories 1455; Niacin 4.96 mg. (approx. 5.0 mg.)
Based on W. Wilson (n. 20), p. 16.

year, as well as those who showed overt symptoms of pellagra at the time of first examination. The last case of pellagra left the hospital in June 1917 and, although there were a few relapses in 1917 and 1918, the disease was virtually wiped out in the camp. Wilson believed that the curative effects of the pellagra preventing properties of the new diet were due to increases in the amount and quality of protein, though analysis of his camp diets shows that this assumption was only partially correct.

Pellagra, as we have learned, is caused by a deficiency of niacin, this term being used in the generic sense for two forms of the vitamin, that is, nicotinic acid and nicotinamide. The vitamin functions in the body as a component of important coenzymes that are necessary to tissue respiration and fat synthesis. Estimation of niacin requirements are complicated by the fact that a fraction of the amino acid, tryptophan, present in dietary proteins, is converted to niacin, and that therefore niacin requirements are supplied both by the protein in the diet and by the dietary content of the preformed vitamin. Proteins of animal origin, that is, milk, eggs, and meat, as well as fish, contain approximately 1.4% of tryptophan while those of vegetable origin contain about 1% tryptophan. In cereals including corn, niacin occurs in bound forms which are not available to the human body. Average diets in the United States supply

TABLE 4. Armenian Refugees' Camp, Port Said. Anti-pellagrous Diet for Sick or Ill-nourished Inmates, Feb. 1917.

Articles of Diet	Daily Amount in gm.	Gross Protein	Available (net) Protein	Biological Value of Protein
Bread (wheaten)	600	40	30	12
Meat (-bone)	42	8.4	8	8
Tripe or fish	60	10.5	9.6	9.6
Eggs (1)	40	4.5	4.4	4.4
Lentils	33.3	8	6.4	3.5
Rice	33.3	2.8	2.2	2
Bourghoul	33.3	4	3.2	1.5
Vegetables	100	1.2	1	.5
Onions	15	.2	.18	.09
Butter	30	—	—	—
Oil	15	—	—	—
Milk (buffalo)	350	19	17.5	17.5
Olives	7	.08	.06	.03
Halva	7	.1	.06	.03
Sugar	60	—	—	—
Jam	14	.5	.4	.2
		99.3	83.0	59.15

Calories: gross, 3143
  available, 3002
Niacin: 12.3 mg.

Based on W. Wilson (n. 20), p. 21.

500 to 1000 mg. or more of tryptophan, and 8 to 17 mg. of niacin. Using these values, the original diet in the Armenian Refugee Camp was deficient both in tryptophan and in niacin, and Wilson's dietary changes actually increased both this amino acid and the niacin content of the diets (Tables 3-5).

Comments and Conclusions

Wilson, without any knowledge of the vitamin, niacin, had, in fact, increased the niacin content of the refugees' diet so as to meet their requirements. This achievement is an example of what should be obvious, namely, that if you are able to recognize that a disease is uniformly associated with a lack of the same foods or foods having the same group characteristics, it may be possible to cure or prevent that disease by addition of the missing items.

The striking similarity in the diets of pellagrins in the different

TABLE 5. Pellagra-preventive diet for healthy adults. Armenian Regugee Camp, Feb. 1917.

Articles of Diet	Daily Amount in gm.	Gross Protein	Available (net) Protein	Biological value of protein
Bread (wheaten)	675	45	34	13.6
Meat (-bone)	42	8.4	8	8
Tripe or fish	60	10.5	9.6	9.6
Lentils	50	12	9.6	5.2
Rice	50	3.7	3.7	3
Bourghoul	50	6	4.7	1.9
Vegetables	150	2	1.5	8
Oil	20	—	—	—
Suet	10	—	—	—
Onions	15	.2	.18	.09
Cheese (skim milk)	12	1.8	1.5	1.5
Olives	7	.08	.06	.03
Halva	7	.1	.07	.03
Sugar	20	—	—	—
Salt	15	—	—	—
		90.6	72.5	43.7

Calories: gross, 2693
    available, 2513
Niacin: 12.9 mg.

Based on W. Wilson, *J. Hyg.*, 1921, *20*, p. 21.

countries in which the disease has occurred is of particular interest. It is, however, of far more importance that these people had little or no intake of fresh meats and other rich sources of niacin and protein. Endemic pellagra is a disease of extreme poverty and has occurred particularly in populations who have been fed rather than those who have fed themselves. To elaborate on this concept fully is beyond the scope of this presentation, but it is important to point out that the vast majority of pellagrins have been sharecroppers or persons confined to institutions or refugee or prison camps. A common denominator has not been what they have eaten, but what they have *not* eaten. They have not eaten food of animal protein origin, nor have they consumed vegetable sources of niacin such as legumes. Endemic pellagra has been eradicated from most countries as a result of economic, agricultural, and social development, especially the ending of various sharecropping systems. Neither Roussel nor Goldberger nor Wilson was able to influence those social conditions which provided the basis for the development of all endemic pellagra, though each in his own way recognized the social characteristics of pellagrins. Indeed, the discovery of niacin itself was not time-related to the complete conquest of pellagra. Pellagra remains a major health problem among the Bantu in South Africa, and it is still quite prevalent in Egypt and in the Deccan Plateau region of India. In these countries and in pockets within our own rural south such as in rural Florida, the disease continues to affect the socially disadvantaged groups who, whether they subsist on maize or millet, cannot afford to obtain a pellagra-preventing diet. While anyone now can cure pellagra with a handful of pills, social progress is hardly measurable if the disease still makes its appearance in the same conditions of misery that have been its background since the first cases were observed among Spanish peasants. The fact that pellagra is prevented by the provision of an adequate diet and historical documentation that this was possible without a knowledge of vitamins was supported by the preventive and curative efforts of Roussel, Goldberger, and Wilson.

Notes

1. G. Casal, "De affectione quae vulgo in hac regione 'mal de la rosa' nuncupatur," *Historia natural y medica de el principado de Asturias: Obra posthuma* (Madrid: Martin, 1762), III, 327-360.

2. G. Strambio, Sr., *De pellagra observationes,* 3 vols. (Milan: Mediolani, 1785-89).

3. D. A. Roe, "The sharecropper's plague," *Natural History,* 1974, *83:* 53-63.

4. Idem, *A Plague of Corn. The Social History of Pellagra* (Ithaca, N.Y.: Cornell University Press, 1973).

5. C. A. Elvehjem et al., "The isolation and identification of the anti-blacktongue factor," *J. Biol. Chem.,* 1938, *123:* 137-149.

6. F.-L. Fanzago, *Memoria sopra pellagra del territorio padovano* (Padua, 1789).

7. G. B. Marzari, *Saggio medico politico sulla pellagra o scorbuta Italiano* (Venice: Parolari, 1810).

8. H. Chick, "The causation of pellagra," *Nutritive Abstracts & Reviews,* 1951, *20:* 523-535.

9. C. Lombroso, *Studii clinici ed esperimentali sulla natura, causa e terapia della pellagra* (Bologna: Fava e Garagnani, 1869).

10. W. C. Sullivan, "Pellagra and the price of corn and maize. Editorial comment on G. Antonini, La pellagra ed il prezza del grano e del mais" (*Arch. di Psichiat.,* 1901, *22:* 202), In *J. Ment. Sci.,* 1901, *47:* 823-824.

11. T. Roussel, *De la pellagre* (Paris: Hunnyyer & Turpin, 1845).

12. P. Thouvenel, *Traité sur le climat d'Italie considéré sous ses rapports phisiques, météorologiques et médicinaux* (Verona, 1797).

13. F. Frapolli, *Animadversiones in morbum vulgo pelagram* (Milan: Galeatium, 1771).

14. J.-M. G. Hameau, *De la pellagre* (Paris: Rignoux, 1853).

15. C. B. Davenport, "The hereditary factor in pellagra," *Arch. Int. Med.,* 1916, *18:* 4-31.

16. L. W. Sambon, *Progress report on the investigation of pellagra* (London: Bale & Danielsson, 1910). Reprinted from *J. Trop. Med. & Hyg.,* 1910, *13:* 18-27.

17. T. Roussel, *Traité de la pellagre et des pseudo-pellagres* (Paris: Bailliere, 1866).

18. A. Bordier, *La geographie médicale* (Paris: C. Reinwald, 1884).

19. A. Marie, *La pellagre* (Paris: Giard et Briere, 1908).

20. W. F. Lorenz, "The treatment of pellagra: Clinical notes on pellagrins receiving an excessive diet," *Public Health Reports,* 1914, *29* (2): 2357-2360.

21. J. Goldberger, C. H. Waring, and D. G. Willets, "The prevention of pellagra: A test of diet among institutional inmates," *Public Health Reports,* 1915, *30* (2): 3117-3131.

22. W. H. Wilson, "The diet factor in pellagra," *J. Hyg.,* 1921, *20:* 2-58; see p. 5.

Discussion

Peter H. Niebyl

Pellagra is a disease that immediately elicits strong feelings of indignation at its existence, too strong to allow for any sense of humor to be intended in the title of Dr. Roe's paper, yet I confess finding irony in any "attempts at the eradication" of anything, especially an historical review of it. Eradication promises a definitive result so often used to justify multiple attempts despite actual failure. Dr. Roe, instead of concentrating on what she implies is the too often touted success of Goldberger, rather seeks to find his predecessors, not his immediate ones, but rather those of earlier centuries. Modern medicine was not the first to relate diet in general, and corn in particular, to the cause of pellagra and our modern medicine may not be the last, since pellagra is still common in some countries and still found here in Baltimore.

Professional claims for expertise in eradication of pellagra vary with the species of experts. Although professionals are all carnivorous, each finds the meat of the problem in a different factor. The clinician-dermatologist tries to establish the specific criteria for the diagnosis. Who has, or really did have, pellagra? Was Casal's collar really a contact dermatitis? The laboratory scientist, on the other hand, wants to specify the biochemical formula for the deficient dietary factor. Even today there is still confusion about the precise crucial dietary factor or factors in pellagra. Needless to say, clinical dietary deficiency of the magnitude seen in pellagra may involve multiple deficiences. On the other hand, it was the historical existence of starvation without pellagra that needed explanation. The social scientist, even when disguised as a social historian, wants to know the specific socioeconomic condition leading to the deprivation. The government bureaucrat—be he from the Hapsburg monarchy or from the administration of southern United States asylums —tries to find the cheapest calories for the masses, corn being an obvious solution. Yet government agent Goldberger solved the problem in the

same southern asylums. The poor epidemiologist, of course, must consider all these factors and more. The clever historian, if he remains pure,
can avoid all these factors content with pointing out a few ironies during
the course of his narrative. Any actual parallel between past and present
is condemned as presentism. Thus it doesn't really matter whether it was
our pellagra that Casal described—period pellagra remains pure. Finally,
the poor patient and the population at risk—the antithesis of the relatively well-fed, well-educated professional and the only group not represented here today—has an even greater vested interest in pellagra
research. They are perhaps the unsung heroes of this disease having
been the first to recognize it, to name it, and to take dietary steps to
avoid it. It took epidemic proportions of the disease to get medical
attention. Otherwise obscure physicians made medical history by simply
listening to and observing their patients—thrust upon them by historical
circumstance. Even Goldberger's research depended on a patient population that could not be found in a teaching hospital much less a university
per se.

Dr. Roe has appropriately blended her own multi-disciplinary background to deal with the complex history of this imposing disease. In her
fine book on pellagra[1] she gives social factors a definite role in her
description of the Hapsburgs' crushing a radical movement whose news-
paper is entitled *Il Pellagroso*. Her emphasis today is on the establishment's more constructive attempts to eradicate pellagra. In her book the
scientific approach takes on the taste of the historian's irony when she
depicts the eminent Davenport, publishing elaborate pedigrees of hereditary pellagra in prestige medical journals. How common it is to both
history of medicine and modern medicine, that every disease gets subjected to the new, emerging—already partly successful—concept of
disease. A good example of novelty's seeming triumph over experience,
no matter how sound, can be found in the description of another vitamin
deficiency disease in Osler's *Modern Medicine* of 1907.[2]

The view has recently been gaining ground that scurvy is the result of a specific
infection which takes place through the mouth. . . . [Victor] Babes . . . succeeded
in reproducing some, at least, of the features of the disease in rabbits by
injecting them with cultures taken from the gums of patients suffering from
scurvy. He demonstrated, also, in the blood of his cases, a bacillus which he
believed to be the cause of the disease.

Even scurvy succumbed to the germ theory of disease. Conversely,
modern medicine now looks on acrodermatitis enteropatrica, once

considered due to a yeast infection and more recently considered a hereditary disease, as now due to a zinc deficiency. If we can indulge in historically based prediction, pellagra and scurvy will perhaps in the near future be considered immunological diseases. These diseases would then lose their purely historical interest and rejoin the modern medical research front. A corollary of any rule that novelty triumphs over knowledge would be that novelty can justify mistakes. Thus one can apologize for Davenport's hereditary pellagra by pointing to the subsequent discovery of Hartnup's Disease—a hereditary error in tryptophane metabolism with pellagra-like symptoms. The clinician, of course, would want to know if Davenport's cases really were cases of Hartnup's Disease.

A feature common to all the various professional research approaches to pellagra was to find a new specific basis for the specific disease, be it genetic, metabolic, or infectious. Ostensibly, George Searcy's article of 1907, even more than the earlier European precursors discussed by Roe, anticipated Goldberger by showing that the nurses who handle the affected pellagrous patient, but do not eat their diet, do not get their disease. Yet like the other precursors Searcy did not consider his finding inconsistent with the notion that the cause of pellagra might be in a damaged, poisonous form of corn that could simply be remedied by pure food laws. They could only see specificity in toxins, poisons and germs. Similarly, an 1881 editorial on pellagra in an American journal, the *Medical Record,*[3] pointed to bad social conditions, especially famine, as a general cause of pellagra, yet at the same time considered contaminated corn as the specific cause and possibly due to a fungus. Dietary deficiency and cure with a proper diet did not conflict with the idea that the specific cause was a toxic factor in the corn. Even Goldberger himself entertained this possibility for a while. But unlike all his clinico-epidemiologic predecessors, Goldberger was also aware of an academic network of scientific publications involving F. G. Hopkins, Osborne and Mendle, Casimir Funk, and E. V. McCollum all of which centered around a narrower concept that was not at all readily evident to clinicians and hospital administrators. This was the idea that the specificity of the clinical syndrome might be due to specificity in the dietary deficiency. This idea was almost as foreign to them as Archibald Garrod's idea that clinical specificity could be found in inborn errors of metabolism. In their search for specificity, toxins and germs had previously appeared the most readily available answer. That is why the latest research on scurvy pointed to bacteria rather than to a specific chemical substance in limes. Once Goldberger grasped the idea that specificity could be found in diet—he set up a conceptual dichotomy between the idea of a specific dietary deficiency and the toxic-contaminated corr theory as alternative explanations for the specificity of the clinical disease—he could then give old data new meaning, e.g. the failure of the nurses to become affected. Although he perhaps failed as a lab man in trying to grind out the specific missing biochemical material, he succeeded in ridiculing the toxic theory. In the case of his "filth parties," where he and his friends ingested the excreta from every orifice of pellagra patients, he was able to show the population at large they would not contract the specific disease in this way.

Pellagra historically had been called the Italian leprosy. Extensive skin disease seems to evoke an almost instinctive fear of filth and contagion. Indeed much of the deep emotional reaction to the thought of pellagra is not only due to its association with the class of people affected but also to the visual effect of extensive skin disease in the severe cases that come to public attention. Even today extensive skin disease often evokes both a general revulsion and a fear of contagion among surrounding patients and even among medical personnel. Perhaps Goldberger's greatest achievement was to fight a deep-seated popular prejudice by grasping a new basis for the specificity of disease hitherto appreciated by only a very small academic group. In this he had few precursors.

The so-called ontological concept of disease—the idea that there are specific disease entities—to some extent has been around ever since the recognition of epidemic disease with characteristic skin lesions plague, smallpox, measles, and subsequently pellagra. Only with the rise of the concept of specificity among professional and research groups did the basis for disease specificity expand as they justified their budgets with attempts of eradications. Fortified research, fortified bread and a fortified economy have all contributed to the partial success.

If I may close on a personal note, I grew up in the small town of Milledgeville, Georgia, where Goldberger did most of his famous work at the State Hospital. I even recall my high school nutrition course. Yet I cannot recall ever having heard about Goldberger or his work. Nor did I hear about it in my subsequent courses in the history of medicine in several northern cities. Perhaps it was too recent to be real history and for that reason Dr. Roe may have been wise to concentrate on the earlier story.

Notes

1. Daphne Roe, *A Plague of Corn: The Social History of Pellagra* (Ithaca and London: Cornell University Press, 1973).
2. Robert Hutchinson, "Scurvy," in William Osler, ed., *Modern Medicine: The Theory and Practice* (Philadelphia and New York: Lea Bros., 1907), vol. 1, p. 896.
3. "The scourge of Italy," *Med. Record,* 1881, *20:* 413-414.

The Germ Theory of Disease

Phyllis A. Richmond

"The Germ Theory of Disease" is the name given to the notion that a living agent of contagious matter might be the specific causal factor in a wide range of transmissible diseases. By "specific causal factor" is meant the environmental factor or "remote" cause—cause outside the body—without which there could be no diseases. Other environmental factors might or might not be present but this factor was necessary for the disease to occur.

The possibility that living matter might seriously be considered in the etiology of diseases had been one of a number of speculations with a long history, generally dating back to the Romans—Lucretius, Varro and Columella—[1]though probably more surely from Fracastoro.[2] It takes considerable care to distinguish between the various views about living contagion. The general feature of reproduction or replication within the human body was a basic requirement and the proposed "germs" were invisible to the naked eye. By the beginning of the nineteenth century, two concepts of *contagium vivum* were postulated: an atomistic one of a substance or specific ferment for each disease, capable of rapid reproduction within the body but apparently lifeless outside of it;[3] the other claimed a minute organism which behaved as if alive outside as well as inside the body. The earliest descriptions referred to little "animalia," "insects" or "animalculae."[4] The clearest expressions of the animalcular concept before the nineteenth century were presented by Giovanni Maria Lancisi[5] and Marcus Antonius Plenciz,[6] the latter being quite explicit both on the nature of such organisms and their individuality, claiming that each disease was associated with a different animalcular agent. Probably there was a parallel development with regard to parasitic diseases such as scabies and favus, not to mention trichinosis.

The animalcular hypothesis in the early nineteenth century was expressed in three different ways. First, living organisms were actually considered to be "little animals," generally similar to protozoa; second, the living matter was of vegetable origin in the form of germs, spores or fungi; third, both kinds of living organisms were accepted, but they were considered to be chemical catalysts and not the exciting cause of the resultant disease. There was also a zymotic theory, similar to the third version, which considered a ferment, or a poison with properties of life, as the agent. Ultimately the first two views merged and the third survived in the concept of a bacterial toxin.

During the first four decades of the nineteenth century, the animalcular hypothesis was refined[7] so that information on the means of transmission, growth and development became available for discussion and the reasoning for proving it was suggested in Henle's Postulates.[8] The actual methodology for proving the germ theory took a long time to evolve. In the first place, scientific terminology was vague. While new concepts bring new words with them, [9] the process moves slowly as a discipline gradually emerges.

Secondly, other scientific developments were helpful. One was research in microbiology, typified by Christian Ehrenberg's study of the infusioria,[10] which included a classification of bacteria and the early use of staining. Agostino Bassi's discovery of a microscopic plant in a disease of silkworms,[11] various observations of microorganisms in conjunction with disease (but without proof as to their relationship), better classification of bacteria, and research on yeasts and fermentation enhanced the numerous theories of disease connected with environmental factors. These theories resulted in a movement to clean up the air and water, dispose of wastes, harness major epidemics such as cholera with barriers (which failed of their purpose) and, in general, to improve hygiene. Major controversies developed over spontaneous generation, contagiousness or noncontagiousness of various diseases, the part played by factors such as night air, polluted air, insects and animals in the production of disease, the nature of sepsis, the part played by man in spreading disease, and so forth.[12]

In the process of gradually developing a more rigorous science, experimentation and the discovery of reliable techniques—experimental work that could be verified every time—became a matter of heartbreaking trial, failure, new trial, new failure, until, by a process amounting to successive approximations, success was achieved. Henle's Postulates were redrawn in scientific terminology as Koch's Postulates. The establishment of the germ theory in the etiology of infectious and communicable diseases was not only a triumph of science, but also a source of several new fields of science, each with its own theoretical basis and rationale, collection of techniques, body of knowledge, trained personnel at all levels, and ultimately a secure position as a scientific discipline with academic respectability. Medicine was able to progress from concern with cure to capability of prevention, which had major ramifications in public health, medical statistics, medical geography and the science of epidemiology.

This brief summary of the rise of the germ theory of disease and its effects—the development of various sciences whose very nature is based on the concept as a foundation—makes the process sound much easier and its ultimate conclusion more obvious and foregone than it actually was. The germ theory, after all, was a pretty far-out concept up until about 1850. And even then it was vigorously opposed by some of the best scientific minds in Europe. Lest we forget how hard it can still be to find and demonstrate the bacterial nature of a disease, we have before us the example of "Legionnaire's disease."[13] And if that is not sufficient to deter overconfidence, the recent program of the mass vaccination against Swine flu should remind us also that one of the greatest features resulting from the establishment of the germ theory, mass preventive measures, carries with it its own price. This last is something that tends to get lost in historical studies unless there is some reason to notice a hidden cost in an otherwise favorable situation. In the course of the acceptance of the germ theory, a number of aspects were recognized that were not consistent with it, and one can only guess at an explanation in many instances.

None of the paradoxes, questions and inconsistent data are unfamiliar. What is, perhaps, less clear is the route for integrating them all in an effort to re-create a general theory of etiology. There are bibliographic problems which make such a synthesis difficult because of means of access in MEDLARS and MEDLINE. No entry is made under "etiology" or under "etiological theory." Instead a subheading "etiology" has to be tacked onto the name of every single disease. The scattering effect is obvious. Apparently there have been few complaints from users about omission of a section where all the diverse views about etiology can be put together for a general systems theory. Perhaps only popularizers[14] attempt such an ambitious undertaking. Or perhaps there are so many etiological factors that synthesis is believed to be virtually impossible.

What would be the components of such a synthesis? Obviously a "shopping list" would be quite lengthy, since it would include such items as: 1. discoveries relating to specific causal factors such as long-term, slow, inapparent and recurrent viruses; 2. research on the immune system in general and auto-immune diseases in particular; 3. the use of drugs as therapeutic agents, still without a clear concept of the causes of the ailment, as in the case of insulin and diabetes, or lithium and manic-depressive psychosis; 4. genetic factors in predisposition, genetic diseases, other diseases that can be related to heredity, such as those which seem to be related to various types of human constitutions; 5. the role of individual idiosyncracy, including allergy; 6. the plain stubbornness of human beings who use tobacco, alcohol, drugs to excess; who do not make use of existing immunizations for disease prevention; who allow religious and other beliefs to interfere with self-preservation; who decline to pay the costs of pure food, pure air, pure water and so forth; 7. the statistical and observational data on ecological and environmental factors compiled by epidemiologists, both to establish etiological agents and to account for the transmission of disease agents.

The germ theory served as a sole paradigm for more years than etiological and epidemiological information would support. As it gradually became clear that the doctrine of specific contagion was not enough to account for the presence or absence of disease, there was a gradual return to an earlier viewpoint calling for multiple causal factors, but on a firm scientific basis. With this broader viewpoint, for example, there are no infectives and no reservoir of susceptibles for genetic diseases, such as Huntington's chorea, Tay-Sachs disease and many others, only the probability patterns in heredity. Even endemic diseases, where communication or transmission factors are a constant, require an explanation more sophisticated than the presence of the microorganism, the means of its transmission and the opportunity for communication. A receptive host is necessary and a collection of conditions that make for receptiveness in the host. Many other variables can be added. Some of these factors are demonstrated in the type of studies by epidemiologists and medical statisticians, while others still await explanation.[15] The method being used to totally eradicate smallpox is not the shotgun approach of mass vaccination, valuable as this technique is, but the rifle approach of locating each case and tracing its contacts. This method obviously would be less helpful in a roaring epidemic, or in a disease with a non-human reservoir. Thus there are various levels of explanation which may be affected by various types of causation, even when dealing with a single disease.

These oversimplifications merely suggest some of the realities facing epidemiologists and others who seek to define cause and effect in disease with some degree of certainty. The germ theory is only a part of the solution, and possibly a very small part at that. One comes down finally to the mathematics of probability in developing models which will approximate reality.

Considering the number and complexity of the problems which appeared to be *against* the probability of the germ theory being the answer to the etiology of much infectious disease, one is driven to reconsider the matter of causes and effects. For a disease to occur, there has to be a number of causes—predisposing, precipitating, perpetuating, proximate—in addition to the presence of a single specific contagion in a virulent state, ready to act as an exciting, initiating or contributing remote cause. In other words, unlike the ideal laboratory conditions under which cause and effect can be demonstrated in animals in a controlled manner and where similarly controlled experiments may be possible with humans, research results tend to be readily extrapolated to human experience by an inductive leap. That is, the discoveries fit the pattern of those humans who, as susceptibles, acquired the disease. The patterns of removal—those who were infected but did not become ill, those who were ill but survived and those who died—also fit. The negative factors in establishing the germ theory—the presence of natural resistance in individuals in an exposed population, the absence of the necessary concomitant factors permitting development of the disease, and certainly the operation of chance—suggest very strongly that one should suspect the presence of empirical hyperbolic distributions in etiological data. What follows herewith is a speculation, which may or may not have validity.

In writing up scientific research, standard procedure calls for a brief historical explanation giving the background of the problem being investigated. The brevity and historical accuracy vary widely, but in general this introduces the basic setting of the investigation being reported. Citations in this part of a paper are to past work of significance, with the implication that if the reader looks up this material, the report to follow will be seen to be a logical consequence as night follows day.[16] Citations in the results/discussion stage also make use of historical data to bolster arguments and conclusions. Thus scientific or medical history has a special use in on-going research. It makes the research appear to flow in normal channels.

Nineteenth-century descriptions of epidemics tended to begin with quite an elaborate set of conditions, such as temperature, unusual weather, and especially extremes or deviations from normal—anything environmental that appeared to affect the population at risk and therefore might be the remote cause of pestilence. The state of the potential victims was also described at some length, including those instances where the victim appeared to be perfectly normal and the disease hit like a bolt from the blue. The general course of the disease or epidemic was described in detail and its termination, if any explanation could be found to account for the end.

From these rather elaborate descriptions, which, before acceptance of the doctrine of specific contagion, were commonplace, one may infer that there was a state of normalcy. Certain epidemics occurred in the winter and others in the summer. Some diseases favored a locale such as swampy lowlands, others, crowded living places. In Europe and North America, a large number of such diseases, particularly the cold weather ones, still are latent in the population. Over a period of time this results in a large number of immunes and probably a number of carriers. The distribution of specific causal factors—microorganisms capable of initiating disease—is widespread. A large segment of the population harbors them. The distribution, therefore, of an endemic disease should be that the vast majority of the population will have been clinical or subclinical cases. Only a minority remains to be infected and this minority decreases as the season progresses. The curve for the annual frequency distribution of such diseases should tend to be hyperbolic (skewed). This "distribution" actually may be of several different kinds: it can extend over time with the long tail representing sporadic cases; it can be distributed over age, with the long tail representing a pool of younger victims; it can be influenced by susceptibility, with the long tail representing increasing resistance as the season wears on, and so on.

In epidemics there is a frequency distribution of a different sort, more like the standard Gaussian curve until the epidemic begins to wane. Toward the end one would expect a hyperbolic distribution. With recurring epidemics, such as cholera in the nineteenth century, the population may self-select, voluntarily or involuntarily, its victims; those who can flee will do so and those who are left become infected in varying degrees. The morbidity and mortality rates accordingly decline.

Similarly, with tuberculosis and several other diseases, a decline in susceptibility or a rise in immunity in the population will tend to replace the Gaussian curve by a skewed one. With some diseases, effective preventive measures also can induce such a change in the pattern of distribution.

The empirical hyperbolic distributions, as represented in the "laws" variously named for Fechner, Zipf, Pareto, Bradford, Willis, Mandelbrot and others, tend to represent social rather than natural causes.[17] An exception has been found in the work of Lewis Fry Richardson on determining the length of coastlines, probably the first indication that the distribution occurs in nature as well. Benoit Mandelbrot has recently introduced a methodology which probably will allow broader usage of it.[18]

The hyperbolic distributions have a unique characteristic—that of self-similarity. Any segment of the curve representing the distribution yields exactly the same pattern as the whole, but on a different scale. This can be demonstrated graphically in instances where the general pattern is repeated in smaller and smaller replications of itself—the scale being the chief factor in making the difference in appearance. The result is an elegant complexity providing more information, but still capable of being re-scaled to a simple pattern of proportionate size. Both scaling up and scaling down can be done without altering the original design. The mathematical process of "tilting the plane" is the special case where the different scalings are contained within a finite region.[19]

Mandelbrot has named the phenomena involved "fractals," defined as "a mathematical set or concrete object whose form is extremely irregular and/or fragmented at all scales." Technically, each curve has a fractional dimension greater than its topological dimension. "A scaling fractal can be defined roughly as any geometrical pattern (other than Euclidean lines, planes and surfaces) with the remarkable property that no matter how closely you inspect it, it always looks the same."[20]

The illustrations in Mandelbrot's book clearly suggest that the type of hyperbolic distribution discussed here is not limited to coastlines. It does not take too lively an imagination to notice that some of the graphic results look like representations of colonies of bacteria,[21] or situations where the process of clustering has been used to describe things like Invisible Colleges.

While this paper was in preparation, an interesting illustration turned up in an unexpected place—the alumni magazine sent to graduates of

the University of Pennsylvania. The work of Robert Austrian in developing a vaccine for the pneumonias caused by the pneumococcus was
described. He reported: "We were able to show that 6 types of pneumococci cause half of the cases, 12 cause three-fourths, 18 cause about
seven-eighths. . . ."[22] Over 80 different pneumococci had been identified
in a study of 4,000 cases. Obviously the disease situation here is an empirical hyperbolic distribution. This is more easily shown with a thousand
case base:

6 types account for ½ of all cases	= 500 cases
6 types account for a further ¼	= 250 cases
6 types account for ⅛	= 125 cases
62 types account for ⅛	= 125 cases

From this it was possible to make a table of simulated experimental
results and derive the typical graph (on plain paper). For 1000 cases, the
results are better if 7 types account for the second ¼, but this would be
in the realm of experimental error, or, if Mandelbrot is correct, of
chance.[23]

This, of course, is just the beginning. From here the methods of
Mandelbrot would be applied to produce much more sophisticated frag-
mental curves as they may occur in nature. Perhaps some of the volumi-
nous medical statistics of the early twentieth century may reveal new
patterns of interest both to historians of medicine and to epidemiologists.
The large number of variables present, in addition to the specific causal
factor elucidated via the germ theory of disease, suggests that a quantum
leap in the level of explanation is needed for full understanding of the
production or non-production of clinical disease. The irregularities of
nature and the need for adequate, less regular, curves for accurate
descriptions of them suggest the use of new kinds of models.[24] Refinement
of such models with the Mandelbrot fractals could add a measure of
form, chance and dimension to the explanation of the role of etiological
factors in disease.

Notes

1. Titus Lucretius Carus, *De rerum natura libri sex,* ed. Cyril Bailey (Oxford: Clarendon
Press, 1947), I, pp. 570-571 (Bk. VI, lines 1092-1102); Marcus Terentius Varro, *Rerum
rusticarum libri tres,* ed. Georg Goetz (Lipsiae: B. G. Teubner, 1912), pp. 26-27 (Bk. I,
Ch. 12); Lucius Moderatus Columella, *On Agriculture, De re rustica,* trans. H. B. Ash
(Cambridge, Mass.: W. Heinemann, 1941), pp. 62-63 (Bk. I, Ch. 5).
2. Girolamo Fracastoro, *De contagione et contagionis morbis et eorum curatione libri*

III, trans. W. C. Wright (New York: G. P. Putnam's, 1930), Bk. I, Ch. 1-13; p. 302; p. 302, n. 5.

3. Jean Astruc, *De morbis venereis libri sex,* in E. R. Long, *Selected Readings in Pathology from Hippocrates to Virchow* (Baltimore: C. C. Thomas, 1929, originally published in 1736), pp. 63-65; James Tytler, *A Treatise on the Plague and Yellow Fever* (Salem: Printed by Joshua Cushing for B. B. Macanulty, 1799), p. 190; Samuel Brown, *A Treatise on the Nature, Origin and Progress of the Yellow Fever* (Boston: Printed by Manning & Loring, 1800), pp. 93-95; Louis B. Guyton-Morveau, *Traité des moyens de désinfecter l'air, de prévenir la contagion, et d'en arrêter le progrès* (Paris: chez Bernard, an IX, 1801), pp. 232-234 (paragraphs 145-146).

4. Charles Singer, *The Development of the Doctrine of Contagium Vivum 1500-1750: A Preliminary Sketch* (London: Privately printed, 1913).

5. Samuel Latham Mitchill, "A translation from the Latin of the celebrated J. Mar. Lancisi's work, De noxiis paludum effluviis," *Med. Suppository,* n.s. 1818, *6:* appendix, 201-212, 311-332, 442-467 (bk. I, ch. 16-19).

6. Marcus Antonius Plenciz, *Opera medico* (sic) *physica . . .* (Vienna: John Thomas Trattner, 1762), 32-44, 55-79 (tractate I, sect. I, ch. 45-47; sect. II, ch. 72-94).

7. John Gideon Millingen, *Curiosities of Medical Experience* (Philadelphia: Haswell, Barrington & Haswell, 1838), 352-353; Jean-Chrysanthe Galés, *Essai sur le diagnostic de la gale, sur les causes et sur les conséquences médicales pratiques à déduire des vrais notions de cette maladie* (Paris: Didot Jeune, 1812); Henry Holland, *Medical Notes and Reflections* (Philadelphia: Haswell, Barrington & Haswell, 1839), 342-355; Jacob Henle, *On Miasmata and Contagia,* trans. George Rosen (Baltimore: The Johns Hopkins Press, 1938).

8. Henle, *On Miasmata and Contagia,* passim.

9. Karl Kisskalt, *Theorie und Praxis der medizinische Forschung,* 2nd ed. (Munich: Lehmann, 1944), 189.

10. Christian Gottfried Ehrenberg, *Die Infusionsthierchen als volkommene Organismen* (Leipzig: L. Voss, 1838). A French translation was attached to Louis Mandl's *Traité pratique du microscope . . .* (Paris: Balière, 1839), pte II, sect. II, 426-427.

11. Agostino Bassi, *Del mal del segno calcinaccio o muscardino* (Lodi: Dalla Tipografia Orcesi, 1835-36).

12. Cf. Phyllis Allen, *Americans and the Germ Theory of Disease* (Ann Arbor: University Microfilms, 1949), for more detail.

13. Cf. "Science and the citizen," *Scientific American,* Feb. 1978: *238:* 80-84.

14. An informal attempt written primarily for laymen may be found in Rene Dubos, *The Mirage of Health* (New York: Harper, 1959).

15. Mervyn Susser, *Causal Thinking in the Health Sciences: Concepts and Strategies of Epidemiology* (New York: Oxford University Press, 1973).

16. Sheila Joan Kelley Bertram, *The Relationship between Intra-Document Citation Location and Citation Level* (Ann Arbor: University Microfilms, 1970). Dissertation no. 70-20, 925. Citations in the title/introduction section proved to be of more recent origin than Bertram anticipated even though they were spread over a greater range of years than in other parts of a paper (cf. pp. 197-209). This may have been unique to the subject studied.

17. Robert A. Fairthorne, "Empirical hyperbolic distributions (Bradford-Zipf-Mandelbrot) for bibliometric description and prediction," *J. Documentation,* 1969, *25* (4), 319-343.

18. Benoit B. Mandelbrot, *Fractals: Form, Chance and Dimension* (San Francisco: W. H. Freeman, 1977), p. 294. In introducing the subject (p. 17) he writes: "Each piece of a straight segment is like a reduced scale version of the whole. . . . Either in a strict or statistical sense, nearly all are *invariant by certain transformations of scale.*" He points out

that the idea is not new, but what is new is that his contribution "is addressed to *geometric* aspects of self-similarity in Nature."

19. Examples may be found in the work of M. C. Escher, e.g. Bruno Ernst, *The Magic Mirror of M. C. Escher* (New York: Ballantine Books, 1976); M. C. Escher, *The Graphic Work of M. C. Escher* (New York: Ballantine Books, 1971); M. C. Escher and J. L. Locher, *The World of M. C. Escher* (New York: Harry N. Abrams, 1973). Also during the past two or three years, commentary appears in the "Mathematical Games" department of the *Scientific American.*

20. Martin Gardner, "Mathematical Games," *Scientific American,* 1978, *238* (4), 21.

21. Mandelbrot, *Fractals,* pp. 214-215.

22. *Pennsylvania Gazette,* 1978, *76* (5), 14-15.

23. See attached appendix for simulated data and raw curves.

24. The simple random walk pattern "approximating a Brownian line to line function and its zero set" has been carried along so that its iterations end up looking almost like a photograph. See Mandelbrot, *Fractals,* plates 214-215, showing "islands" which could represent the results obtained by cluster techniques or bacterial growth. Plates 210-211 look like landscapes of the moon and elswhere sent back by satellites.

Discussion

Alfred S. Evans

Dr. Richmond has presented a brief summary of the rise of the germ theory from her extensive knowledge of the subject. She has then given us a "shopping list" of items that might help create a more general theory of etiology, emphasizing the difficulties in classification and nomenclature in library retrieval systems, such as Medlars in obtaining data on the multifactoral origin of diseases. These include information on the agent, immune system, drugs, genetics, host response, and host behavior. She has dealt with the number and the complexity of factors contributing to causation and stressed that the organism is a necessary but usually insufficient cause of disease. Dr. Richmond then pointed out that the annual distribution of certain endemic diseases is skewed—in regard to number of cases, the age of the patients, and the diminishing pool of susceptibles. She calls this skewed distribution "hyperbolic."

In the final portion of her presentation Dr. Richmond discussed Mandelbrot's "Fractals" and their application to the discovery of new patterns of etiology. It is here that Dr. Richmond and I part intellectual company. I have read the reference she says is the most clearly written account of the subject—a paper by Fairthorne[1] entitled "Empirical Hyperbolic Distributions (Bradford-Zipf-Mandelbrot) for Bibliometric Description and Prediction." I did understand *one* statement: "the same social phenomena may have several different causes, acting severally or in concert." However, the conclusion left me gasping for breath, i.e., "This survey has shown the hyperbolic distribution to be the inevitable result of combinatorial necessity and a tendency to short-term rational behavior whenever a group of people have to use a repertory of given elements to form compounds, and when one aspect of the "cost" or inconvenience of these elements is dominant." After much search in Yale's libraries, I finally found a copy of Mandelbrot's recent book *Fractals: Form, Chance, and Dimension.*[2] Again, most of this fascinating

94

TABLE 1. Technical Developments and the Discovery of Microbial Causes of Disease

Development	Examples
1. *Light microscope*	*M. Leprae*
2. *Laboratory Animals*	
Guinea pig	*M. Tuberculosis*, Legionnaires' Disease
Ferrets	Influenza
Adult mice	Herpes simplex, yellow fever
Suckling mice	Coxsackie, newer arboviruses
Chimpanzee	Hepatitis B, Kuru, Creutzfeldt-Jakob
Armadillo	Leprosy
3. *Bacterial Culture* (agar culture)	Most bacteria
4. *Embryonated eggs*	Herpes, smallpox
5. *Tissue Culture*	
Monkey kidney	Enteroviruses, Lassa
Adult human	polio, adeno, RS
Embryonic human	
Lung (WI 38)	CMV, rhinoviruses, corona virus
Cord lymphocytes	EBV
Brain	Papova (JC strain)
6. *Electron microscope*	Hepatitis A, rotavirus
	EBV
7. *Fluorescent antibody*	*M. Pneumoniae*, etiology of I.M.

book was over my head. Professor Cochran warned us today of "the danger of reading thoughts and books to which we are not equal." I will, therefore, leave the field of forms and fractals entirely to Fairthorne, Mandelbrot, and Dr. Richmond and say a few simple words of my own.

Most advances in our knowledge of causes of disease have not come in a quantum leap because some genius developed a new theory or performed a magnificent intellectual feat. Rather, they have evolved as a result of technical advances and simple good luck—sometimes termed serendipity. Such discoveries are often not the result of premeditation or design and are based on an adventitious or unexpected phenomenon, sometimes not included in the original research plan. Table 1 presents some of these technical developments and some of the discoveries that have been based on them. Every time a new instrument—a light, electron, or scanning microscope is developed, new etiological agents are found. In recent years the demonstration of the Epstein-Barr virus, hepatitis A and B viruses, and rotaviruses were made with the electron microscope. Every time a new experimental host is used, new agents are isolated. The introduction of various tissue cultures resulted in the isolation and identification of a whole plethora of new viral agents.

TABLE 2. Evolution of Concepts of Causation in Infectious Diseases

Concept	Date	Person
Bacteria as cause of infectious	1840	J. Henle
disease	1890	R. Koch
Viruses as cause of infectious		
disease	1937	T. Rivers
Epidemiologic proof of causation	1957	R. Heubner
Multiple causes of same syndrome	1960	A. Evans
Immunologic proof of causation	1968	W. Henle, A. Evans
Slow viruses as cause of	1974	R. Johnson and C.J. Gibbs
neurological diseases		
Viruses as cause of cancer	1974-76	G. Miller, A. Evans, M. Epstein
Immunological processes as	1959	E. Witebsky
cause of disease	1962	B. Waksman

TABLE 3. Henle/Koch Postulates of Causation

1. Causative agent present in every case of disease and under circumstances to account for pathological changes and clinical course.
2. Causative agent occurs in no other disease as fortuitous and nonpathogenic parasite.
3. Causative agent can be isolated in pure culture, passed repeatedly, and induce the disease anew in experimental model.

Koch, R., 10th Int'l. Congress, Berlin, 1890.

Proof of Causation

The elements necessary to prove that a given organism is responsible for causation of a given condition also varies with the technology available at the time. Table 2 presents a chronological summary of the main historical events in the evolution of these concepts of causation and I have discussed them in detail elsewhere.[3] They began with the ideas of Jakob Henle in 1840 which were elaborated by Robert Koch in 1890 (Table 3). These Henle/Koch postulates have been used to guide us ever since but unfortunately have many limitations some of which were recognized by Koch at the time they were presented, and others recognized as new technology for identifying infectious agents developed. For example, Koch recognized that the causes of cholera, leprosy, diphtheria, typhoid fever and relapsing fever, could not fulfill all the criteria he outlined. Later discoveries of the healthy carrier state, of viruses, of the multifactoral causation of disease, of agents that could be cultivated in the laboratory (EB virus, hepatitis viruses), or those which also produced no immune response (Kuru, Jacob-Creutzfeldt),

TABLE 4. Limitations of Koch's* Postulates of Causation

1. Not applicable to all pathogenic bacteria.
2. May not be applicable to viruses, fungi, parasites.
3. They do not include the following concepts:
   a. The asymptomatic carrier state
   b. The biologic spectrum of disease
   c. Epidemiological elements of causation
   d. Immunologic elements of causation
   e. Prevention of disease by elimination of putative cause as element of causation
   f. Multiple causation
   g. One syndrome has different causes at different settings
   h. Reactivation of latent agents as cause of disease
   i. Immunological processes as cause of disease.

*More properly termed The Henle-Koch Postulates.

TABLE 5. Steps in Discovery of Causation of Infectious Diseases

	Examples
1. Serendipitous or purposeful discovery	
a. In the laboratory	Pencillin, EB Virus and IM (infectious mononucleosis)
b. In the clinic	Rubella and congenital malformations
2. Retrospective analysis of characteristic (microbial agent) in cases and controls	Many viral diseases
3. Prospective study of incidence of disease in presence or absence of characteristic	EBV and IM
4. Removal or modification of characteristic or its means of transmission to prevent the disease in controlled trial	Typhoid transmission Immunization: polio, smallpox

each required revision of the criteria for causation. Similarly, the contribution of viruses to the pathogenesis of cancer and the multifactoral role of etiological agents involved in chronic diseases spurred additional guidelines of causation as well as an effort to draw together a "unified concept" for both infectious and non-infectious diseases.[4] Thus, over the 138 years since Jakob Henle first put forth his ideas and almost 90 years since Koch presented his postulates many limitations to their application have appeared which are outlined in Table 4 and discussed in a recent letter to the *Lancet*.[5] We have now recognized that the steps in unraveling the role of a putative causative agent in a disease involves not only the isolation of the agent and microbial proof but also epidemiological proof (Table 5). Because of the complexity of this interplay of multiple factors, one of the most impressive demonstrations of the importance of the agent is a decrease in the incidence of the disease when the putative factor is removed or modified. We can all take refuge in the fact that effective control of disease does not wait on absolute proof of causation. By identifying and modifying the means of transmission of the agent, or breaking some other link, or removing a cofactor involved in the pathogenesis of the disease we may achieve effective control without full recognition of the nature of the cause.

Notes

1. Robert A. Fairthorne, "Empirical hyperbolic distributions (Bradford-Sipf-Mandelbrot) for bibliometric description and prediction," *J. Documentation,* 1969, *25:* 319-343.

2. Benoit B. Mandelbrot, *Fractals: Form, Chance, and Dimension,* 1st ed. (San Francisco: W. H. Freeman, 1977).

3. Alfred S. Evans, "Causation and disease. The Henle-Koch postulates revisited," *Yale J. Biol. & Med.,* 1976, *49:* 175-195; idem, "The Parran Lecture—causation and disease. A chronological journey," *Amer. J. Epidemiology.*

4. Evans, "Causation and disease."

5. Alfred S. Evans, "Limitation of Koch's postulates," *Lancet,* 1977, *2:* 1277-1278.

The History of Smallpox Eradication

Donald A. Henderson

On October 22, 1977, a 23-year-old hospital cook living in the southern Somalian town of Merka developed high fever and headache.[1] He was hospitalized and treated for malaria but the symptoms persisted. Four days later a rash developed. Chicken pox was suspected and he was discharged home to recuperate. By the fifth day, it was apparent that the disease was not chicken pox but smallpox and this was subsequently confirmed by the laboratory. Investigation revealed that on 13 October he had been exposed to two cases of smallpox—at that time the only known active cases in Somalia. The cook in turn had exposed 161 persons, 41 of whom were unprotected. All were identified, vaccinated and kept under surveillance. None developed smallpox.

During the following six months, more than 3,000 Somali, Ethiopian and Kenyan health staff, assisted by some thirty World Health Organization (WHO) advisors, searched systematically village by village throughout the Ogaden desert and adjacent areas.[2] In Somalia alone, more than 6,800 cases of rash with fever were each investigated by national and international teams. More than 500 specimens were examined by the WHO Smallpox Reference Center at the Center for Disease Control in Atlanta. None were smallpox. Further assurance that smallpox transmission has been interrupted was provided by a survey conducted throughout Somalia during March and April 1979. The survey revealed that 70% of the adults knew that there was a substantial reward for reporting a smallpox case and knew where to report a case. The reward accounts, in part, for the large number of suspect cases reported.

What may ultimately be the world's last case of naturally acquired smallpox, Ali Maalin, became ill in October 1977. In Ethiopia, no cases have been discovered since August 4, 1976. Since that date, all known cases of smallpox have been in Somalia except for 5 in Kenya during January 1977, resulting from an importation from Somalia. Documentation sufficient to demonstrate conclusively that transmission has been interrupted in all previously endemic areas is still required. Such programs are in progress and should be completed in 1980.

Conceptually, the eradication of smallpox could be said to date back to 1801. That year, three years after he performed his classic experiment demonstrating that cowpox infection protected against smallpox, Edward Jenner wrote: "it now becomes too manifest to admit of controversy that the annihilation of the Small Pox, the most dreadful scourge of the human species, must be the final result of this practice [of vaccine inoculation]."[3] Jenner's statement is better characterized as enthusiastic hope rather than a feasibly imminent achievement. Although the practice of vaccination was rapidly disseminated around the world, provision of supplies of vaccine and their satisfactory preservation proved difficult. The production of vaccine in quantity was not achieved until the mid to late 1800s when cowpox-vaccine virus began to be produced by growth on the flank of a calf.[4] In the 1900s, the increasing availability of refrigeration assured better preservation of the vaccine. Finally, developments in cryopreservation culminated in techniques which permitted production of a highly stable freeze-dried vaccine preparation. By 1940, many European countries with a temperate climate and advanced health delivery systems had become free of smallpox during the course of intensive, compulsory vaccination programs.[5] Outbreaks which occurred were controlled by the isolation of patients and mass vaccination. Epidemiological studies provided considerable information in regard to patterns of smallpox transmission but little practical use was made of this knowledge in national programs. Program strategy consisted essentially of mass vaccination. The possibility that smallpox might be eradicated over a large geographic area was subject to speculation but was not seriously considered.

The proposal that smallpox eradication over a defined geographic area be undertaken as a definitive public health objective dates back only to 1950. Dr. Fred Soper, then director of the Pan-American Sanitary Bureau (PASB), proposed that a program for eradication be undertaken throughout the Americas.[6] Soper was an articulate proponent of disease eradication programs, an interest which originated from his work with the Rockefeller Foundation's Yellow Fever Commission. Efforts to eradicate yellow fever from the Americas had commenced in 1915 at the instigation of Dr. William Gorgas. Gorgas had shown in Havana that the reduction of *Aedes aegypti* breeding resulted in the disappearance of yellow fever. In 1909, he boldly expressed the view that eradication of the disease could be achieved by temporary anti-aegypti campaigns in key-endemic centers. The Rockefeller Foundation supported this effort in Brazil and a campaign was begun, hopefully to be completed in five to ten years.

The difficulties and the costs proved more formidable than had been anticipated. Gradually, the objective shifted to eradication of the *Aedes aegypti* mosquito species itself, the urban vector of yellow fever. Remarkable successes were achieved in the Rockefeller-supported Brazilian program but reinfestations from neighboring countries regularly occurred.

Immediately following World War II, Soper became director of the Pan-American Sanitary Bureau and in 1947 its governing body approved a resolution granting for the first time to an international health organization responsibility "for coordinating the activities of a number of countries in the permanent solution, through eradication, of a regional health problem."[7] Although *Aedes aegypti* eradication has yet to be achieved, the resolution set a precedent for Soper's next proposal, in 1950—the eradication of smallpox throughout the Americas.

The principal strategy then and the strategy which dominated national smallpox control and eradication programs through 1966 was mass vaccination. The stated objective was to vaccinate 80% or more of the population in each country. It was anticipated that when this was achieved herd immunity would result in cessation of virus transmission.[8] Control measures of varying intensity were implemented when outbreaks occurred, but systematic efforts to improve reporting systems so as to detect cases promptly and to contain all known outbreaks was not part of the strategy. The elementary but important principle that smallpox spread in an identifiable continuous chain with one infected person transmitting the disease to another was understood but essentially ignored in program execution. Recognition of this principle dictated a strategy which was designed to contain each outbreak, each link in the chain of infection, and through identification of sources of infection to detect outbreaks which might not have been reported but were still persisting. Illustrative of the lack of appreciation of the basic epidemiological behavior of smallpox was the frequent reference by many otherwise competent epidemiologists to the occurrence of "sporadic" outbreaks and cases. That each case invariably constituted but one link in a continuing identifiable chain of transmission was all but ignored.

As recently as 1967, reporting was so incomplete that in most areas, not more than one percent of all cases were being reported.[9] Official

morbidity data are thus of limited value in tracing the historical incidence
and spread of smallpox. In the United States itself, official records of the
National Office of Vital Statistics show "sporadic" cases reported by
state and local health officials for fully six years after the last documented
case in 1949.[10] Not until 1955 was it decided that every reported case
must be definitively investigated by state and federal health officials.
The problem was little different elsewhere. In a number of countries,
such as those in the western Pacific and Central America, successful
programs were conducted in the 1950s and 1960s.[11] However, data regarding the occurrence of cases are so incomplete and fragmentary that
it is impossible to determine when smallpox transmission was actually
interrupted.

Employing the strategy of mass vaccination, eradication campaigns,
begun in the Americas in 1950, succeeded during the succeeding eight
years in interrupting smallpox transmission in the Carribean, in Central
American and in certain of the South American countries. On the global
scene, however, WHO and many of the developing countries were fully
preoccupied with another Soper-inspired and largely American-financed
malaria eradication effort. The magic of the comparatively new and
inexpensive insecticide, DDT, had resulted in rapid interruption of
malaria transmission in southern Europe and in pilot projects in Asia
and the Americas.[12] National programs had little more than started when
it was discovered that certain mosquito strains were beginning to show
resistance to DDT. Responding to this, the World Health Assembly
decided that WHO should embark on an intensified global campaign to
eradicate malaria before resistance became widespread. The effort
demanded prodigious resources, a national and international commitment, reasonable political stability in the infected countries and a high
degree of organization and management. The task was formidable.

In 1958 the Soviet Union offered an alternative program to the
American-dominated malaria eradication campaign. At the World Health
Assembly, its delegates proposed that there be a global commitment to
undertake smallpox eradication.[13] A definitive resolution was passed the
following year. The plan envisaged a two-year period to produce sufficient stocks of vaccine. This was to be followed by an intensive globally
coordinated three-year vaccination program. Principal funding was
expected to be through voluntary donations from the developed countries
who were at risk of smallpox importations. Voluntary contributions
were solicited but an average of less than $100,000 per year was received
in cash and in kind. A number of countries undertook mass vaccination
programs but the results were disappointing. An Expert Committee was

convened by WHO in 1964 to assess the situation.[14] Although acknowledging that improved notification was desirable to assess smallpox incidence, the Committee's dominant concern was vaccination. This is exemplified in its conclusion: "The continuing recurrence of smallpox in areas where the vaccination program had been completed was proof that many remained unprotected." The Committee concluded that "the target must be to cover 100% of the population." In brief, there was no more than passing reference to the epidemiological characteristics of smallpox transmission, or to an alternative strategy which might be more effective.

Concern increased as the program of smallpox eradication continued to founder. Finally, the World Health Assembly requested the Director-General to prepare a special report indicating what was needed to achieve smallpox eradication. He proposed that WHO be granted some $2 million per year in supplemental funds to help coordinate and finance a global program and that voluntary contributions be substantially increased.[15] The proposal was welcomed by many but viewed skeptically by most. Failures in the eradication of yellow fever and subsequently of the *Aedes aegypti* mosquito in the Americas and a foundering malaria eradication program did not recommend yet another eradication program.

With less than universal enthusiasm, the WHO Smallpox Eradication Program commenced in January 1967. The strategy proposed in WHO's Field Handbook, published in July 1967, continued to emphasize the importance of systematic vaccination programs which focused initially on cities, towns and villages which were noted to "represent the most important reservoirs of the disease."[16] The important difference between the strategy before 1967 and the strategy thereafter related to the addition of epidemiological surveillance as a principal component. The use and application of epidemiologic surveillance in disease control programs had been well demonstrated during the 1950s by Langmuir and his colleagues at the U.S. Public Health Service's Communicable Disease Center.[17] Surveillance programs began with malaria, diphtheria and poliomyelitis and subsequently were extended to deal with many other disease problems. Application of the technique to smallpox eradication was a logical extension. The Smallpox Program's Field Handbook stated as follows:

It is necessary for the eradication programmes to develop a systematic plan for the detection of possible cases and the concurrent investigation regarding the source and site of acquisition of infection, their vaccination status and the prompt instigation of containment measures. Detailed epidemiological investigation of all cases as to the reason for their occurrence and the means by which they are being spread can be one of the most effective instruments to provide continuing guidance and direction to the vaccination program. In the simplest terms, each case which occurs suggests the possibility of flaws in the program. . . . Even in countries with limited local health services, a systematic surveillance plan can and must be developed as an essential component. . . .

It was thought initially that it would require not less than two years to develop a satisfactory surveillance scheme to permit prompt reporting, investigation and control of outbreaks. Moreover, it had been assumed that such measures would be of limited effect until smallpox incidence fell to levels of perhaps 1.0 case per 100,000 population or, in smaller countries, to less than 100 cases per year. Thus, it was planned to undertake first systematic programs of vaccination which would reach 80% of the population. The figure of 80% was selected as an operationally achievable standard. This strategy was soon altered. Eastern Nigeria provided a first indication that effective reporting systems could be developed in a matter of months rather than years and that transmission could be interrupted in a population with a comparatively low level of immunity and an incidence higher than 1.0 case per 100,000. Foege, then serving as an advisor in eastern Nigeria, initiated a reporting scheme based principally on a radio network linking mission health stations.[18] Vehicles and other supplies for the program had not yet arrived and so, utilizing available resources, he undertook intensive containment vaccination in areas from which cases were reported. The source of infection of the first case in each outbreak led to the discovery of other outbreaks. Within months and before a systematic vaccination campaign could be started, transmission was interrupted. Vaccination scar surveys revealed that not more than half the population had ever been vaccinated, a level of immunity far lower than what had been anticipated to be required before surveillance containment measures could be effective. More than this, it was apparent that less than 5% of all cases had occurred in persons who had ever been vaccinated. This suggested that vaccine efficacy ratios, even after 10 to 20 years, were far higher than had been expected, an observation later confirmed by more detailed studies in other areas.[19] Lastly, it was apparent that even though the incidence was high, the cases were concentrated in groups of villages and, within the villages, were clustered geographically. This reflected the need for close contact between individuals for virus to be transmitted between the infected person and susceptible contacts. The comparative ease with which outbreaks could be stopped indicated that even in a densely populated, developing country, smallpox spread more slowly than had been anticipated. Rarely did the infected person transmit the disease to more than 3 to 4 additional persons. Additional studies were conducted in other countries of west Africa[20] and Brazil[21] and these confirmed that the Nigerian observations pertained there as well.

Accordingly, the strategy was altered to stress that primary emphasis should be given to the development of surveillance-containment measures from the inception of all programs. Systematic programs of vaccination, however, were to continue to reduce the number of susceptibles and cases and so facilitate the surveillance-containment measures. Country program directors and international advisors were so instructed but only limited success was achieved in altering the strategy. It was soon apparent that the supervision and resources required to implement systematic vaccination programs preempted both manpower and material. Little remained which could be diverted to surveillance-containment activities. Only by deliberate overemphasis of the importance of surveillance-containment activities did changes begin to occur. Not surprisingly, custom and tradition sustained the vaccination component of the campaign.

Recognition that even a single vaccination confers effective protection over one to two decades led to a second shift in strategy. Primary vaccination was stressed with the admonition that, except in outbreak containment, revaccination was unnecessary. Again, this overstated the true situation since immunity gradually wanes over time. However, the change in strategy led program directors to focus their attention on less well-vaccinated segments of the population rather than repeatedly revaccinating the most accessible groups, such as school children, in order to increase their totals of vaccinations performed. In consequence, overall protection materially improved.

In most of Africa, in South America and in Indonesia, comparatively modest efforts to improve reporting and fairly simple containment measures sufficed. On the Indian subcontinent, however, comparable efforts were not successful.[22] Program organization and management were problematical but there were epidemiological factors as well. Population densities were far greater than in most of the other areas and vaccination immunity levels only marginally better. The net effect was that the density of susceptible persons was higher. A second factor was the greater degree of population movement. The Indian subcontinent has a relatively extensive network of railroads and a large population which travels by railroad, by boat and by bus, few of whom purchase tickets. Large numbers of lower socioeconomic people, often unvaccinated and sometimes infected with smallpox, thus traveled frequently and over long distances from rural villages to urban centers and back. A third problem was the plethora of religious festivals, each attracting hundreds of thousands to millions of persons.

In June 1973 the strategy again was altered to address these problems. More rapid and complete case detection was achieved by mobilizing in India more than 100,000 health workers for a monthly week-long village-by-village later house-by-house search for cases. Special surveillance-containment teams (fire fighting teams) were mobilized and trained to deal with each outbreak which was discovered. More rigid containment procedures were employed which required watch guards to be assigned to each infected residence and teams were assigned to live in the villages to vaccinate the ever-numerous population of visitors. Finally, a reward was offered to those reporting cases. This system was soon extended throughout the adjacent countries. Less than two years elapsed between inception of this strategy and the occurrence of the last case in Asia on August 16, 1975.

The final stronghold of the disease was the eastern horn of Africa, among nomads who roam the vast Ogaden desert. In other areas populated by nomads, such as in the Sahel of West Africa or Afghanistan, it had been found that endemic transmission did not long persist among the nomad bands themselves. The number of susceptibles in each nomad group and the limited contact between groups usually resulted in spontaneous interruption of transmission within a few generations of disease. In the Ogaden, there was yet one more unexpected finding. In contrast to West Africa or Afghanistan, where case fatality rates were 10% to 25%, the disease in the Ogaden was exceptionally mild with a case fatality rate of less than 0.5%. Even those in the acutely ill phase were mobile—remarkably mobile. During the rainy season of 1977, for example, when roads were literally impassable to vehicles, workers commonly covered 60 kilometers or more during a 24-hour period, often walking at night. Unfortunately, the patients did also. Moreover, the disease spread less readily from patient to contact. Among those with the more severe forms of variola, there was a direct correlation between severity of disease and facility of spread. The rule applied also in the Ogaden. Many instances were documented among nomad groups in which smallpox persisted for 4 to 6 months among small groups with only one or two cases in each generation. The virus and the population had achieved a remarkable equilibrium. Containment of outbreaks was also a more difficult problem since the Ogaden nomads moved erratically and without warning from area to area, in contrast to Afghani or Aahelian nomads whose pattern and timing of movement was far more predictable.

Techniques for case-detection and control which gradually were adopted were a cross between those used previously in Africa and Asia. Progressively, through tight control of populated areas and constant search for cases and containment, literally on a catch as catch can basis, smallpox incidence declined until finally on October 26, 1977, the last known case of naturally acquired smallpox occurred.[23]

These, in outline, were the principal events in the historical evolution of smallpox eradication from its inception through the successful execution of the program. The introduction of epidemiological surveillance, translated from its previous form at CDC, proved ultimately to be the key to success. Only the broader shifts in strategy are described; numerous other more subtle modifications in strategy and tactics could be illustrated.

From the experiences of the last 10 years of the campaign, it was all too apparent that however much we felt we knew about smallpox and its behavior before the global program began—and we knew a great deal —we learned much, much more during its execution. Essential was a better understanding of the epidemiology of the disease and it was this which dictated continuing change both in strategy and tactics. Comparatively few of the studies and observations were sufficiently detailed to meet the rigid standards required for publication in scientific journals. There was neither time nor manpower for carefully randomized studies nor time to document all facets of each of the investigations, but observations of varying degrees of sophistication served repeatedly to alter the course of the program nevertheless. I am confident that a far closer relationship than now exists between active programs and epidemiological study could have a comparable salutary effect on many other programs now in progress.

Notes

1. Joel G. Breman, "Smallpox: No hiding place," *World Health,* August 1978, pp. 24-29.

2. World Health Organization, "Smallpox surveillance," *Weekly Epidemiological Record,* 1978, *53:* 125-131.

3. Edward Jenner, "The origin of the vaccine inoculation," in: E. M. Crookshank, ed., *History and Pathology of Vaccination* (London: H. K. Lewis, 1889), vol. 2, p. 274.

4. Leslie Collier, "The preservation of smallpox vaccine," *Trends in Biological Sciences,* 1978, *3:* 27-29.

5. C. W. Dixon, *Smallpox* (London: J. & A. Churchill, 1962), pp. 463-464.

6. Pan-American Health Organization, *Handbook of the Governing Bodies* (Washington: Pan-American Health Organization, 1970), p. 27.

7. Fred L. Soper, "The elimination of urban yellow fever in the Americas through the eradication of *Aedes aegypti,*" *Amer. J. Public Health,* 1963, *53:* 7-16.

8. World Health Organization, *Expert Committee on Smallpox,* Technical Report Series, No. 283 (Geneva, 1964).

9. Donald A. Henderson, "Smallpox eradication," *Proc. Royal Soc. London,* 1977, *199:* 83-97.

10. Dixon, *Smallpox,* p. 467.

11. Ibid., pp. 466-469.

12. Lloyd E. Rozeboom, in: Maxcy-Rosenau, *Preventive Medicine and Public Health,* ed. by Philip Sartwell 10th ed. (New York: Appleton-Century-Crofts, 1973), pp. 436-439.

13. World Health Organization, *Official Records, No. 87 of the 11th World Health Assembly* (Geneva, 1958), pp. 508-512.

14. WHO, "Smallpox eradication."

15. World Health Organization, *Official Records, No. 152 of the 19th World Health Assembly* (Geneva, 1966), pp. 258-296.

16. World Health Organization, *Handbook for Smallpox Eradication Programs in Endemic Countries* (Geneva, 1967).

17. A. D. Langmuir, "The surveillance of communicable diseases of national importance," *New England J. Med.,* 1963, *268:* 182-187.

18. W. H. Foege, I. D. Miller and J. N. Lane, "Selective epidemiologic control in smallpox eradication," *Amer. J. Epidemiology,* 1971, *94:* 311-318.

19. Donald A. Henderson, "Eradication of smallpox: The critical year ahead," *Proc. Royal Soc. Med.,* 1973, *66:* 493-500.

20. Foege, Miller and Lane, "Selective epidemiologic control in smallpox eradication."

21. C. C. de Quadros, L. Morris, E. A. Costa, N. Arnt and C. H. Tigre, "Epidemiology of variola minor in Brazil based on a study of 33 outbreaks," *Bull. World Health Org.,* 1972, *46:* 165-171.

22. M. I. D. Sharma and N. C. Grassett, "History of achievement of smallpox 'target zero' in India," *J. Communicable Diseases,* 1975, *7:* 171-175.

23. Breman, "Smallpox: No hiding place."

Discussion

Genevieve Miller

It is a remarkable coincidence that smallpox, the first disease which man began to protect himself against through an active medical procedure, is also the very first to have been eliminated from the earth. It would almost seem that this has been a demonstration over the past 250 years of the great wisdom which science engenders whereby man is enabled to proceed rationally towards desired goals because of an ever increasing knowledge of nature. While science-engendered progress is undoubtedly true in many instances, the victory over smallpox is marked throughout much of its history by a lack of basic scientific knowledge. The victory actually came as the consequence of a pragmatic approach rather than from guidelines originating in scientific thought. In fact, one can show a number of instances in which attempts to give scientific explanations actually retarded progress, with only practicality and common sense restoring the fight against smallpox to its ultimately successful course.

In reviewing the history of the conquest of smallpox it is important to emphasize in the beginning that Jenner's introduction of vaccination was not necessarily the crucial step towards the ultimate victory that has commonly been assigned to it, for seen in the larger picture of the counterattack against smallpox which began in the first decades of the 18th century, Jenner's contribution appears as a sensible modification of an already well-established prophylactic procedure, rather than as a complete innovation. Thus this discussion will include comments on variolation as well as vaccination, because success with the former was an essential antecedent of the latter.

In an earlier publication I have discussed in detail the introduction of variolation, an empirical folk practice of Africa, the Middle East, and China into Western Europe, particularly Britain and her colonies.[1] It was introduced, not for the simplistic reason that Lady Mary Wortley

Montague had her daughter inoculated with smallpox in London during an epidemic in the spring of 1721, but because for years the mounting horror of smallpox which nearly everyone contracted sooner or later stimulated the medical and scientific community to seek new remedies. Sydenham had modified its treatment from warming to cooling procedures to make the patient more comfortable. When reports came to England of actual preventive measures in other parts of the world, whether of blowing powdered smallpox scabs into the nose as the Chinese were doing or of applying matter from a smallpox pustule to a scratch in the skin as was being done in Turkey, the scientific community which centered in the Royal Society of London was very much interested and actively sought further information which in turn was widely discussed and published. Even if Lady Mary had not had her daughter inoculated, Cotton Mather and Boylston in Boston would have introduced the practice of inoculation to the western world, since their efforts were carried out independently without knowledge of Maitland's inoculation of the Montague child. The knowledge of the practice combined with the fear of the disease inevitably would have led to trials, and the actual individuals who did try inoculation first are not causative agents in a major sense.

General accounts of the history of smallpox have overlooked the efforts of members of the Royal Society to have experiments performed to assess the result of variolation and to serve as a clearing house for information, just as a generation later in France the Académie Royale des Sciences with the encouragement of the *philosophes* explored and promoted the new practice. It was the scientists who produced convincing statistical evidence of the value of inoculated smallpox in reducing the chances of death from the disease. In spite of occasional setbacks the popularity of the practice grew from a small number of inoculations among the aristocracy in the 1720s to become widely practised among all classes in England by the end of the century.

Peter Razzell's recent books argue very convincingly that "smallpox had virtually disappeared as a disease amongst the wealthy classes by about 1770, which . . . can only have been due to the practice of inoculation."[2] He produces evidence that the increase in the population of England during the latter part of the century was directly caused by the decline in smallpox mortality, as many contemporary writers also observed. Jenner's substitution of relatively harmless cowpox for smallpox virus in the inoculation procedure eliminated the basic objections of a possibly fatal outcome or that inoculation might spread the disease.

Razzell however casts a shadow on the much celebrated role of Jenner by attempting to prove that although the original Jennerian experiments were with true cowpox virus, his later vaccine which was distributed widely in England, Europe and around the world was actually derived from smallpox "and that the bulk of the vaccine used for the first forty years or so of the nineteenth century was an attenuated strain of smallpox virus."[3] Even today the relationships of the three viruses of variola, cowpox, and the vaccinia currently used in vaccination are not clearly understood. Electron microscopic and chemical structural analysis reveal no differences among them. Neutralization and complement fixation tests with antigens prepared from these viruses show a serological overlap. According to Downie, their identification in the laboratory depends upon "differences in host range, the appearance of the lesions produced on the chick choriollantois, their rate of growth in tissue culture, and their ceiling temperatures."[4] We do not even know the origin of the vaccinia virus currently used in vaccination which is produced in laboratories by scarification of the skin of calves and sheep. Some believe it was derived from variola virus attenuated through continuous passage in human skin, others that it is a hybrid derived from simultaneous human infection with variola and cowpox, and others believe it is a laboratory virus derived from natural cowpox by continuous artificial propagation.[5]

These comments serve to illustrate my introductory comment that much of the final victory over smallpox was achieved without precise scientific knowledge. Smallpox was overcome because a certain procedure worked. Let us now examine some of the instances in which attempts to link scientific theory with the battle against smallpox actually retarded its progress.

When inoculation was originally introduced in the early eighteenth century, the most common medical theory about smallpox was that expressed in the tenth century by Rhazes, who first described the disease and followed classical humoral theory by placing its seat in the blood. Every person was born with something in the blood, variously described as an innate ferment, seeds, contagion, virus, or venom which at some time in his life had to be expelled through the skin. This, of course, explained why everyone succumbed to the disease, and why children tended to have milder cases since they had not yet acquired habits of intemperate living and other blood-corrupting agents. The early London inoculators, believing that an incision in the skin would facilitate the expulsion of the innate disease-causing agents, used a lancet to insert the virus and in many cases made deep incisions through the skin, unlike the light needle scratches of the Greek women in Turkey. A plaister was then applied. This procedure tended to put the virus directly into the blood stream and produced more severe cases.[6] Only later did they begin to realize that a light scratch was sufficient, for the best results were obtained when the incision did not go through the skin.

Similarly influenced by their humoral theory, the early inoculators established a routine preparatory period in order to establish the optimum condition for the blood to receive the smallpox virus. Impurities were supposedly removed by bloodletting and purging, as well as by special diets. Periods of from three to four weeks of such preparation often endangered patients exposed to natural smallpox epidemics before their inoculation, and in numerous instances patients had themselves inoculated sooner to escape the disease in the natural way, only to succumb to the natural smallpox before the inoculated form had taken effect. By the 1760s several inoculators began to advertise inoculation without preparation, a method popularized by the Suttons who inoculated thousands without harm, by essentially reverting to the original folk method of inserting the virus in a slight scratch in the skin without any preliminary preparation. In 1767 a trial experiment with the Suttonian method on 74 children in the Foundling Hospital in London averaged a little more than 20 pustules per case, a much smaller number than earlier reported cases. In addition the Suttonian method required the use of "unripe, crude or watery matter" from the early stage of development of a smallpox pustule when the infectious material was less virulent.

When Jenner substituted cowpox for smallpox virus in the operation, he believed erroneously that cowpox vaccination would produce permanent immunity. This error, though recognized soon on the continent, survived until the last decades of the nineteenth century in England. In 1889 the Royal Commission on Vaccination argued that infant vaccination gave lifelong protection except in very unusual circumstances. Until the development of precise knowledge of immunological mechanisms in the body, even the compulsory vaccination of children continued to be a debatable issue. However, in spite of all the errors introduced by faulty theory, preventive prophylaxis continued, largely by the accumulation of empirical evidence of its effectiveness.

The history of the victory over smallpox also illustrates the progressive evolution of institutional means to control disease. In the beginning years of inoculation only the wealthy and their servants were given protection. If one were inoculated at home, the fees were high, and care in a private inoculation house for from 4 to 6 weeks was only possible for the upper classes. Soon charitable institutions such as the Smallpox and Inoculation Hospital in London, founded in 1746, became a model for others in the provinces to give free inoculations; in the country wealthy noblemen frequently paid the local surgeon to inoculate their tenants. By midcentury when a smallpox epidemic broke out in a small village, it was not uncommon for the entire non-immune population to be inoculated at parish expense. In time of war the general inoculation of troops began as soon as the disease appeared, as happened with Washington's army during the siege of Boston in 1775. Towards the end of the eighteenth century societies for the inoculation of the poor sprang up in Britain and her American colonies. There was frequent controversy because of the danger of spreading smallpox through inoculation, but the plan developed in 1778 by John Haygarth for an Inoculation Society in Chester, which provided a general inoculation every two years for the non-immune children of the poor, was carried out with careful isolation of the patients and handling of the infectious material. Similar societies were formed in Leeds and Liverpool. In fact Haygarth formulated a plan to eradicate smallpox entirely from Britain by these means.

After the introduction of vaccination, the service through institutions continued at centers in London like the Smallpox and Inoculation Hospital, the Royal Jennerian Society, and the Vaccine Pock Institution. Outside London the Newcastle Dispensary which had been giving free inoculations from at least 1786 changed to vaccination. Some communities offered parents a half crown to have their children vaccinated. It has been estimated that in cities like London, Glasgow, Newcastle, and Manchester probably one-half of the infants were vaccinated during the early years of the 19th century. Some people mistrusted vaccination and preferred to be inoculated. The extensive smallpox epidemic from 1837 to 1840 in Britain activated legislation against inoculation and provided for state-paid vaccination for children of the poor. The Act of 1853 made vaccination of all infants before the age of 3 months compulsory but was not enforced effectively.

Rulers of continental nations were quick to initiate vaccination as a substitute for the increasingly popular inoculation. Napoleon mandated compulsory army vaccination; by 1801 it was practiced in 105 towns in France. In Spain in 1803 King Carlos IV sent a Royal Maritime Vaccination Expedition to his colonies in Mexico, Guatemala and the Philippines to initiate the practice there. Because of the difficulty of delivering active virus at such a great distance, the infection was transmitted by serial vaccination of twenty-two male orphans ranging in age from three to nine years.[7] In Russia Czar Alexander had vaccination performed throughout his empire. In general government regulation developed slowly, and serious epidemics occurred until the present century. By the beginning of the twentieth century most western countries had a partially immunized population within which smallpox epidemics could be checked by mobilizing vaccination facilities through public health agencies. By midcentury the disease had virtually disappeared from the advanced countries of the world and, as we have heard, the final assault became possible through international organization and planning of the World Health Organization. Even here empirical results modified the original strategy. The original goal of vaccinating 80 percent of the population in countries with endemic smallpox was modified when an inadequate supply of vaccine required a change in plan and the discovery was made that the campaign could be carried out successfully by only searching out cases and vaccinating contacts and others in the immediate area. Smallpox was wiped out of some areas with as few as 6 percent of the population actually vaccinated.

While it is entirely coincidental that the first disease for which prophylactic immunization was developed is also the first to be wiped out, one is reminded of the joyful optimism of the eighteenth-century author of the article on smallpox inoculation in the *Encyclopédie* who labelled it the most beautiful discovery ever made in medicine for the conservation of human life.[8] How delightful that the story has a happy ending.

Notes

1. Genevieve Miller, *The Adoption of Inoculation for Smallpox in England and France* (Philadelphia: University of Pennsylvania Press, 1957).

2. Peter Razzell, *The Conquest of Smallpox: the Impact of Inoculation on Smallpox Mortality in Eighteenth Century Britain* (Firle, Sussex: Caliban Books, 1977), p. 151.

3. Idem, *Edward Jenner's Cowpox Vaccine: The History of a Medical Myth* (Firle, Sussex: Caliban Books, 1977), p. 5.

4. Allan W. Downie, "Smallpox," in Stuart Mudd, ed., *Infectious Agents and Host Reactions* (Philadelphia: W. B. Saunders, 1970), p. 491.

5. Ibid., p. 493.

6. Razzell, *Conquest of Smallpox*, pp. 6-8, 38.

7. Michael M. Smith, "The 'Real Expedición Marítima de la Vacuna' in New Spain and Guatemala," *Trans. Amer. Philos. Soc.*, n.s., vol. 64, pt. 1, 1974.

8. *Encyclopédie*, t. 18 (Berne & Lausanne, 1782), p. 803.

Yellow Fever: From Colonial Philadelphia and Baltimore to the Mid-Twentieth Century

Theodore E. Woodward

In 1951, the United States Army assigned me to Bermuda to investigate an epidemic of dengue fever. I had received the specific lot of yellow fever vaccine which resulted in my developing hepatitis. Thus began my interest in yellow fever, which was further reinforced by having some letters come into my possession regarding some of the historical aspects of this disease.

Of all the epidemic diseases prevalent in the American colonies, yellow fever provoked the greatest fear. There was considerable debate among colonial physicians regarding the mode of spread of yellow fever. Benjamin Rush of Philadelphia, the leading physician of that era, was a leading proponent of the concept that yellow fever was contagious, which was accepted by many physicians because of his prestige. However, there were physicians particularly in Baltimore, with different views on the manner of spread and method of treatment of yellow fever.

Rush held that yellow fever became contagious under unfavorable conditions resulting from heat, moisture, and organic decomposition.[1] After investigating the outbreak in Philadelphia in 1793, Rush declared that the epidemic had been introduced by putrid coffee unloaded on the docks from a vessel. He noted several cases in which the coffee had supposedly produced fever on the same day it was unloaded.[2]

Briefly, these were the theoretical bases and practical application in which Rush took so much pride and for which he gained the enmity and scorn of many colleagues. The illogical nature of a method of treatment which invariably produced general debility to relieve "excitement of blood vessels," supposedly a result of debility, seems never to have occurred to him.[3]

The frequent outbreaks of yellow fever in the colonies wiped out entire families and caused general panic. Of special interest were the classic epidemics in 1793 and 1794 in Philadelphia and those in Baltimore in 1794, 1797, 1798, 1799, 1800, 1808 and 1819. The Baltimore epidemic in 1797 delayed the outfitting and commissioning of the Constellation.[4]

In 1819, the quarantine imposed by the city authorities of Philadelphia against the residents of Baltimore caused considerable controversy. David M. Reese, a respected physician of the city, described the 1819 epidemic and condemned this particular grievance upon the Port of Baltimore:

> Instance the act of non-intercourse passed by the city of Philadelphia during the late visitation of Baltimore by a distressing calamity. The fact cannot be too severely censured nor too energetically deprecated. They go to show the irremediable injury to social enjoyment and familiar intercourse which the same principle would effect if pursued and practised. It is a cause, therefore, in which no tongue should be silent, no pen idle, nor no individual unconcerned. The cause of science, of philosophy, of humanity, of truth, all are interested in the extermination of this relic of ignorance and superstition. I call upon all governors and legislators, all teachers of philosophy, all votaries of science, all friends of truth, to unite in the destruction of this bane of commercial prosperity, this common enemy of liberty and philosophy.[5]

Furthermore, Reese was highly critical of those who held the doctrine of contagion, particularly

> the civil authorities of the city of Philadelphia, a city which should last of all inculcate such absurdity since that city produced by a few years since a luminary of science whose bright lustre of character has not been extinguished with the lamp of his life, but which will shine with splendor and grandeur when his persecutors shall sink beneath the surges of a dark oblivion. Yes, the spirit of Rush looks down with grief to see science prostrated, and truth sacrificed at the shrine of ignorance and superstititon.[6]

Before Rush died in 1813, he had abandoned his old harsh and unbending view of contagion to the following extent: "Yellow fever is not contagious in its simple state . . . it spreads exclusively by exhaltations from putrified matters which are diffused in the air" and not by contagion conveyed directly from one person to another.[7] However, Reese distinguished between the concepts of infection and contagion. He considered diseases to be infections if they could be contracted by one or more exposures to a "noxious atmosphere" or the "effluvia arising from putrifaction." The term "contagion" was applied to a "specific quality of a malady by which it may be communicated from a sick to a healthy body, by the latter inhaling the breath of the former or by actual contact."[8]

Following Philadelphia's action, the authorities in Virginia and Wilmington, the Mayor of Alexandria and even Annapolis prohibited any intercourse with Baltimore. Ironically, Rush's contemporaries and successors derided him when he renounced the doctrine of contagion. It is true that in the late eighteenth and early nineteenth century, Baltimore did attempt to quarantine itself from Philadelphia and other eastern cities where and when yellow fever was present. This position was changed by the teachings of Potter and Davidge, Baltimore's two respected medical leaders, against the concept of spread from person to person or contact.

Nathaniel Potter, who was a private student of Rush at the time of the 1793 epidemic in Philadelphia, returned to Baltimore later that year and attended patients there and in Caroline County, Maryland. His keen clinical and epidemiologic observations convinced him that yellow fever was not contagious between persons. He communicated his opinions to Rush on 20 August 1793 and again on 28 October 1793. Potter later described the epidemic in Caroline County and stated:

Those various forms of bilious fever, unquestionably owe their existence to the putrifaction of matters on the surface of the earth, after an uncommonly wet spring, followed by the driest and hottest summer that can be remembered by the oldest inhabitants of the country. Whatsoever may be the result of controversy so warmly agitated in your city, respecting the contagion of yellow fever; the epidemick has no pretensions to that character, in any of its forms. The dysenterick form is considered contagious by popular consent, but (me judice) is no more entitled to the epithet contagious, than the remittent or intermittent fevers. With all possible deference to your superior judgment, I cannot prevail upon myself to believe that any fever, arising from vegetable decomposition, is contagious. The origin you have assigned to the epidemick fever of your city is the only one that is physically possible, and therefore you place your adversaries on equal ground with you, by acknowledging the fever contagious. Deny the existence of contagion as unphilosophical, and you've cut them off from every resource. If we admit one of the fevers from marsh effluvia to be contagious, we are bound (a priore), to admit them all to be so; intermittent, remittent, and dysenterick.[9]

Potter, who considered himself the only person in America to deny the contagious nature of yellow fever, requested Rush to publish these views in his paper describing the Philadelphia epidemic of 1793. This proposal was declined by Rush who stated his firm belief, "that all diseases arising from marsh miasmata were contagious in a degree proportional to their malignity, and that the opposite doctrine was utterly untenable."[10]

Potter presented the following views regarding the quarantine laws against Baltimore:

There cannot be a more flagrant or more lamentable proof that the framers of these laws were destitute of every ray of knowledge of the true qualities of contagion, than the exemption of smallpox from the provision of their quarantine laws. That disease which assails our bodies through every sense but one, whose concentrated poison can be preserved for years, which ocular demonstration has proved to have been transported to every part of the commercial world, is permitted to scourge mankind, while we are legislating against a phantom, against a superstition, against a compound of fear and imagination, heightened by a mixture of the marvellous, as fabulous as any of the tales comprehended within the complicated machinery of the heathen mythology. The visions of contagion stand on a parallel with the calculations of judicial astrology, solemn exorcisms, enchanged castles, and the spells of wizards and witches. The age of chivalry is not gone.[11]

Potter attempted to "prove" his point by soaking towels in the "perspirable" matter of a patient with yellow fever whom he had attended on 20 September 1797 and tied them around his head and retired. He reported that in spite of "extreme nauseous fetor" he slept until 7 a.m. with no later incapacitation. In 1798, Potter inoculated himself with "perspirable matter" from a patient who was in the last stages of yellow fever. From other malignant cases, he inoculated himself with suppurative matter from inguinal buboes on 11 October 1798, experiencing only local redness at the inoculation site.[12] Potter's courageous but ill-conceived self-studies really did not prove anything since he was either immune from a prior attack of yellow fever or his test patients did not suffer from the disease or had eliminated the virus from their tissue.

Potter became the first Professor of Medicine at the University of Maryland in 1807. In 1818 he summarized his life experiences and those perceptive observations that he had recorded during outbreaks of yellow fever in Maryland in a classic monograph.

The first printed criticism of the contagious nature of yellow fever was by Potter's colleage, John Beale Davidge, the founder of the University of Maryland School of Medicine and its Professor of Anatomy and Dean. Davidge was a practical epidemiologist as well as a general practitioner. His experiences at Baltimore's harbor areas of Fells and Locust Points convinced him of the non-contagious nature of yellow fever and were first reported in the Federal Gazette of Baltimore on 30 November 1797. These ideas were later reaffirmed, enlarged and embodied in a monograph.[13] Potter's and Davidge's clinical descriptions of yellow fever, like other keenly observant clinicians of the colonial era, were remarkably good.

A young University of Pennsylvania medical student deserves recognition. Stubbins Ffirth, like Potter, went to extremes to contradict the contagious concept. Ffirth, during the epidemics of 1802 and 1803 in Philadelphia, deposited black vomit and blood into incisions made on his arms and legs. He administered black vomit to animals and also inhaled the fumes of six ounces of bloody material which he heated over a sand-bath in a small room: the residue he made into pills and swallowed.[14] Failing in this, he inoculated himself with bloody serum, saliva, perspiration, bile and urine and finally concluded that yellow fever was neither infectious or contagious. Ffirth, like Potter, was courageous, reckless and probably immune to yellow fever. Otherwise, these patients had a disease other than "yellow jack." Deveze, who arrived in Philadelphia from the West Indies in 1793 to participate in the control of the epidemic, also held to the non-contagious nature of yellow fever.[15]

The early writings and studies of Potter and those of Davidge and Potter from 1793 to 1798 clearly establish their priority of authorship concerning the non-contagious nature of yellow fever. The contagious-non-contagious controversy continued throughout the nineteenth century and required a century for its resolution. However, the convictions of these men did suggest important leads.

The observations of colonial physicians in Baltimore, Philadelphia and elsewhere were remarkably accurate concerning various aspects of yellow fever. They were aware of the seasonal incidence of the disease, which occurred between the summer and fall equinox and disappeared with the arrival of the frost. Low ground was not safe whereas high ground was favorable; a sharp wind could increase the areas of disease occurrence in that direction. Persons who visited ill persons during the daytime were spared while a visit at dusk between certain hours often resulted in their developing the disease. Those who had suffered prior attacks were immune. Native negroes from the Caribbean Islands were unlikely to become ill and colonials from the North or immigrants from Europe were at high risk. It is uncanny that Thomas Drysdale, a physician and quarantine official of Baltimore, informed Rush in a series of letters written in 1794 that "locusts were not more numerous in the reign of Pharaoh, than mosquitos through the last few months" (i.e. the epidemic summer session). "Yet, these insects were very rare only a few years past when a far greater portion of Baltimore was a marsh."[16] These observa-

tions were collectively so close to the fact that yellow fever was transmitted by insects such as a domesticated mosquito.

Another Baltimore physician, John Crawford, was prophetic in his
introductory academic address in 1811 when he predicted a relationship
between insects and human illness:

It is not alone in our fields of our gardens that they commit their ravages, they
attack us in our houses, our goods, our furniture, our clothes, our poultry; they
devour the grain in our storehouse, they pierce all our woodwork, they do not
spare us even ourselves.[17]

He further proposed:

I shall then proceed to consider the cause of suffering in the animals that are in
the nearest connexion with us, continue my inquiries through all of the animal
tribes down to the smallest insect, as far as the means of information have been
within my reach . . . so with men, the plague, yellow and every other fever and
every other disease we experience, must be occasioned by eggs inserted without
our knowledge into our bodies.[18]

Napoleon Bonaparte received one of his major defeats on the wings
of the white-legged *Aedes aegypti* and its yellow fever virus. In repelling
a black rebellion in Santo Domingo in the spring of 1802, about 40,000
French soldiers, sailors, officers and civilians, including his commanding
officers and brother-in-law, General Leclerc, died of yellow fever. The
native adversaries were solidly immune to yellow fever by virtue of
having had a prior attack. In January 1803, the impulsive and disgruntled
Napoleon renounced Louisiana because the swamps in the Caribbean
Island had defeated his Legions. He sold to President Jefferson's two
startled emissaries, Livingston and Monroe, the entire area of Louisiana
for fifteen million dollars.[19]

Throughout the nineteenth century, outbreaks of yellow fever continued in the United States, occurred during the summer, ceased with
the onset of frost, favored the southeastern, southern and Gulf Coastal
cities and eluded explanation. Cities that were hardest hit included New
York, Philadelphia, Baltimore, Norfolk, Charleston, Memphis, Galveston, and New Orleans. The last yellow fever epidemic in the continental United States was in New Orleans in 1905; there were 3,384
cases and 443 deaths, nearly all in the "old town." The sporadic outbreaks
which occurred in Baltimore in 1800, 1808, 1819, 1854 and 1876 began
usually at Locust and Fells Points after ships docked from the Indies.

Areas of Baltimore west of Jones Falls and on high ground seemed to possess strange powers of safety.

Among the proponents of the possible insect transmission of yellow fever was Josiah C. Nott, of Mobile, Alabama.[20] He published an essay in which yellow fever was described as a disease that was distinct from malaria. He also refuted the miasmatic doctrine and suggested that both yellow fever and malaria were of insect or animalcular origin.

The Microbiological Era initiated by Pasteur and Koch in the 1880s provided the stage for the solution of the yellow fever enigma. Foritified with the observed clinical and epidemiological facts, scholarly physicians with roots in Philadelphia and Baltimore, played major roles. Recognition must first be given to Carlos Finlay of Cuba, who graduated from Jefferson Medical College in 1855. As early as 1881 he proposed that the mosquito Culex fasciatus (now known as *Aedes aegypti*) was the link in the transmission of the disease. Unfortunately, he failed to confirm these suspicions. The epoch making contribution of the Second Yellow Fever Commission, directed by Walter Reed, is a proud historical achievement. However, several others merit recognition whose contributions are less well known. among them an unheralded scholarly epidemiologist and a courageous clinical bacteriologist.

Henry Rose Carter is relatively unknown as a participant in this dramatic story, although Reed acknowledged his contribution which guided the Commission to success where Finlay had failed. Carter, born in Caroline County, Virginia, fractured his leg after graduation from the University of Virginia, and changed from an engineering career to medicine. He enrolled in 1873 at the University of Maryland Medical School and graduated in 1878 at the age of 26. After interning at its University Hospital, he joined the United States Public Health Service with ultimate assignment to a district of Marine Quarantine Service which embraced several islands and ports in the Gulf of Mexico. Skeptically, Carter questioned the one hundred year old explanation that the agent of yellow fever was conveyed by fomites, contaminated by direct contact with the primary case. For twenty years, he recorded his observations of outbreaks of yellow fever aboard ships arriving at ports in the Gulf Islands and observed a pattern on ships which left South American ports. He noted that one or two primary cases occurred within a day or two of embarkation followed by an interval of two or three weeks and a cluster of new cases. Such clustering was not reported by crews whose voyages lasted less than two weeks.[21] He observed that no yellow fever occurred among baggage inspectors working in the Gulf district who unpacked and inspected baggage from such ports, such as Vera Cruz, Havana and Santiago, where yellow fever occurred frequently. He reviewed quarantine records dating back through 120 years. In 1897, Carter contracted yellow fever and recovered.

In 1898, two years before the dramatic report of the Reed Commission, Carter investigated household outbreaks of yellow fever in Orwood and Taylor, two small towns in northern Mississippi, and concluded that an "extrinsic incubation period" was required for the human transmission of the agent. The following event described in his original paper is a typical example of how Carter's "shoe leather" epidemiological observations strengthened his concept of an extrinsic incubation period:

Mr. S. W. G. of Orwood, was stricken on August 1, remaining in his household for the duration of his illness. Among eight people visiting him between 6 August and 16 August there were no cases of yellow fever; among 34 people visiting him thereafter, there were 33 cases.[22]

After making many similar observations, Carter stated:

The material leaving the patient must undergo some change in the environment before it is capable of infecting another man. The time required for this change is the time of extrinsic incubation.[23]

Transferred to Havana in 1899 to reorganize its quarantine service, Carter met Reed and his team which began its task in June 1900. He kept in close touch with Reed and Lazear, who were already familiar with his Mississippi studies through reports which he had sent them.[24] Reed himself expressed the importance of Carter's work to the Commission's studies. "You (Carter) must not forget that your work in Mississippi did more to impress me with the importance of an intermediate host than anything else put together."[25] Carter had estimated the extrinsic incubation period to be 10 to 17 days, the Reed group set it at 9 to 16 days.

Sir Ronald Ross, who had incriminated the Anophelene mosquito as the vector of malaria, appreciated the significance of Carter's work and recommended him, along with Finlay, for the 1904 Nobel Prize in Medicine.[26] Recognition and honor were bestowed on Reed, Finlay and Lazear but not on Carter or, in full measure, to the next contributor.

James Carroll, born at Woolwich, England, on June 5, 1855, emigrated to Canada at the age of 15, entered the United States Army and, while a soldier in 1886-1887, began the study of medicine in New York. He transferred to the University of Maryland School of Medicine receiving his degree in 1891. For two years he undertook postgraduate work in pathology and bacteriology, which included training at the Johns Hopkins Hospital. He met Walter Reed in 1893, during an assignment to the Army Medical School in Washington. They were associated for the next six years, until 1899, when Surgeon-General Sternberg formed the Second Yellow Fever Commission with Walter Reed (Director), Carroll (second in command) and Jesse Lazear and Aristede Agramonte, who were already in Cuba, as members. Reed and Carroll sailed from New York on June 21, 1900, and reached Havana on the 25th. Reed returned to the United States on August 4th, leaving Carroll in charge of the field work.

Unquestionably, Walter Reed was the dynamic and talented leader of the historical drama which incriminated the mosquito, but Carroll shouldered a lion's share of the work without which the mission's objective may have failed. Based on his strong capability in bacteriology, his initial work with Reed disproved Guiseppe Sanarelli's view that *Bacillus icteroides* caused yellow fever. The small group pursued the mosquito concept which Finlay had failed to confirm. They worked amicably with Finlay throughout their trials. Lazear, the team's entomologist, made allowance for a suitable incubation period in mosquitos, after they had been fed on yellow fever patients. On August 27th Lazear placed on Carroll a mosquito which had been in incubation for 12 days. In four days, Carroll suffered a severe non-fatal attack; it is of interest that the nurse wrote in her notes, "He is delirious, he said a mosquito caused his illness." He recovered and became the first experimentally infected case in history. The views of all non-contagionists such as Potter and Davidge, were now confirmed.[27]

The letter in Figure 1 (from the original) written by Reed to Carroll describes some of the drama of this event.

Surgeon-General Sternberg later commented that "the incubation in the body of the mosquito was probably Reed's idea, and work along that line caused the first successful case—Carroll's case."[28] Tragically, about two weeks after Carroll's recovery, Jesse Lazear died of yellow fever on September 25, 1900. It was not clearly known how he was infected. It is thought that he was infected while on the wards. The following letter from Reed to Carroll expresses his grief.[29]

Washington, D. C.
September 26, 1900

My dear Carroll:
Major Kean's cable, telling of poor Lazear's desperate condition, was quickly

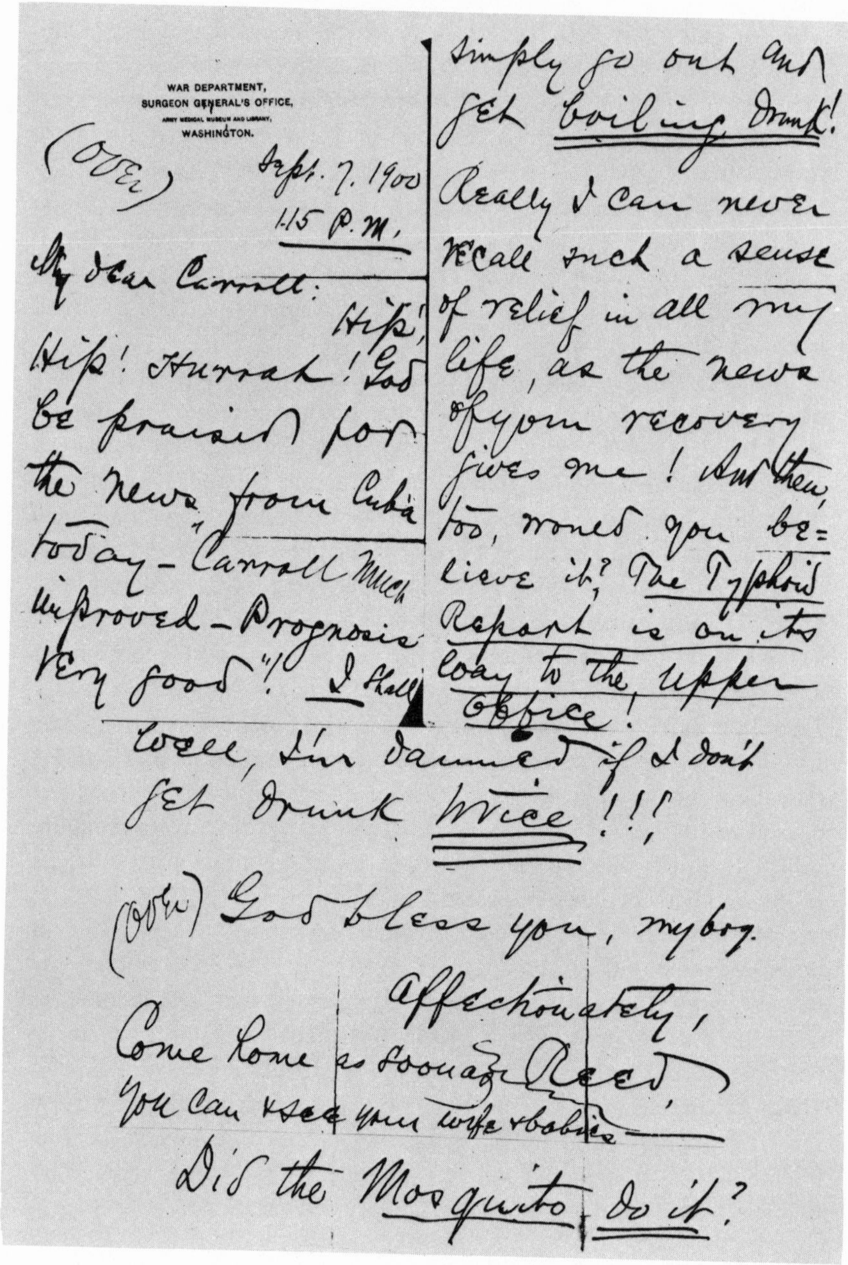

WAR DEPARTMENT,
SURGEON GENERAL'S OFFICE,
ARMY MEDICAL MUSEUM AND LIBRARY,
WASHINGTON.

(Over)

Sept. 7. 1900
1.15 P.M.

My dear Carroll:

Hip, Hip! Hurrah! God be praised for the news from Cuba today—"Carroll much improved—Prognosis very good"! I shall simply go out and get boiling drunk! Really I can never recall such a sense of relief in all my life, as the news of your recovery gives me! And then, too, would you believe it? The Typhoid Report is on its way to the upper Office! Well, I'm damned if I don't get drunk twice!!!

(Over) God bless you, my boy.

Affectionately,
Reed.

Come home as soon as you can & see your wife & babies.

Did the Mosquito do it?

FIGURE 1. Letter, Walter Reed to James Carroll, dated 1:15 p.m., 7 September 1900, on occasion of news of Carroll's recovery.

followed by the one announcing his death—I cannot begin to express my sorrow over this unhappy termination of our colleague's work!

I know that your own distress is just as acute as my own—He was a brave fellow and his loss is one that we can with difficulty fill. I got the general to cable yesterday about securing Lazear's notes which he wrote that he had taken in each case bitten by mosquitoes.—Examine them carefully and keep all.

I will leave here in the morning for New York—and will ask you to meet me with a conveyance at the foot of O'Reilly Street or at the Navy yard dock if you can find out from Quartermaster where passengers will land on the arrival of the Crook, which should be Wednesday, October 3. If your observations are such as you and Lazear have intimated, we must publish a preliminary note as soon as it can be gotten ready.

Affectionately,
Reed

Lazear was born in Baltimore. After graduation from the Columbia University of Physicians and Surgeons in 1892 he spent two years at Bellevue Hospital, New York, followed by training in Europe, including a period at the Pasteur Institute, Paris, and served as Assistant Resident Physician at the Johns Hopkins Hospital, 1895-1896. In February 1900, Lazear was appointed Acting Assistant Surgeon of the United States Army and was assigned to laboratory duty at the Columbia Barracks, Quemados, Cuba. During March and April, Walter Reed spent time in Lazear's laboratory while visiting Cuba.[30] Because of his past experience with mosquitoes in his work with malaria, Lazear was assigned to insect studies.

Carroll continued to be in charge of the field studies until Reed returned to Cuba, again for a short period from October 3 to October 13, and later from November 8 to February 3, 1901. During this period, Reed directed the studies in which Pvt. Kissinger developed induced yellow fever after being bitten by several mosquitoes which had been contaminated by feeding on patients 15, 19, and 22 days previously. Also, during this period, the classic work in volunteers was performed which showed that clothing, bedding and discharges of yellow fever patients were not infectious.

In the summer of 1901, Welch had suggested to Reed the possibility that the infectious agent was filterable based on studies of Loeffler and Frosch on foot and mouth disease of cattle.[31] Such studies were initiated by the Commission.

The use of volunteers for the studies in Cuba became a sensitive issue because in 1901, Finlay and his associate John Guiteras, while conducting vaccine studies in volunteers, independently of the Reed team, encountered two deaths. They and the public became alarmed. Reed, then in Pennsylvania, became disturbed by the exaggerated reports which reached him through the press and on 23 August 1901 wrote Carroll, who was busy recruiting volunteers, conducting the clinical screening and performing the microbiologic and entomologic studies, as follows:

You say 'prospects favorable.' And this leads me to strongly advise against further experiments on humans. Our work has been too good to be marred now by a death. As much as I would like to know whether the filtrate will convey the disease, I shall advise against it.

Carroll however, did not accept this advice and continued with the inoculations of filtered material. He wrote Reed on 22 August 1901 to keep him informed of his plan to continue.

About a week later, Reed responded on 27 August 1901, in which he reversed his views and advised that observations be limited to injection of serum alone without injecting controls with unfiltered blood. The following is an excerpt from a letter from Reed to Carroll dated 27 August 1901:[32]

I wrote you a few days ago advising against further experiments on human beings, in view of these fatal cases. From the tenor of your last letter, however, I see that you have made all preparations to go ahead with the observations as determined by us at Washington, and I hardly know what to say. I will suggest, that inasmuch as the injection of the blood has given us four positive results, you limit your observations to the injections of serum without making controls injected with unfiltered blood.

Sincerely yours,
Walter Reed

After further reflection Reed decided it unwise to interfere with Carroll's plans and cabled him on 29 August 1901.[33]

Consult Havard [Major, Chief Surgeon, U.S. Army]. Use your own judgement in the future.

Reed

Carroll did complete his study and showed for the first time that the causative agent, present in the serum of yellow fever patients, was capable of passing through a filter which excluded bacteria and that the agent in the blood was heat labile (i.e. heated blood from patients was non-infectious for volunteers). After completion of the studies, on 24 October 1901, Carroll answered a reprimand which he had received from the Army Adj. General of Cuba.[34]

Hospital Las Animas
Havana, Cuba

October 24, 1901

To the
  Adjutant General
  Headquarters, Dept. of Cuba
  Havana, Cuba

Through the Chief Surgeon, Department of Cuba

Sir:

   I have the honor to acknowledge the Receipt of Letter dated October 23, 1901 prohibiting any further experimentation among United States troops or civilian employees with yellow fever serum, and conveying the censure of the Department Commander for practicing such experiments upon Privates Hamann and Covington and permitting them to remain with their command "under no restrictions," and beg to submit the following statement:

   Through the courtesy of the Chief Surgeon, Major Valery Havard, I have . . . (In the text of his letter Carroll explains that he had received permission to conduct the experimental studies through appropriate channels, that the command was not placed at risk, nor was serious illness anticipated in the volunteers). . . .

   I am glad to be able to report that my work is completed and I have no desire to make any further inoculations. The results are of inestimable value.

   Of thirteen persons experimented upon, Hamann and Covington are the only ones in the service of the government.

Very respectfully
Your obedient servant
James Carroll
Contract Surgeon, U.S. Army

General William C. Gorgas utilized the findings of the Reed Commission and conquered yellow fever in Havana by the isolation of yellow fever patients and the eradication of *Aedes aegypti* mosquitos. This made it possible to complete the Panama Canal which opened in 1914. With him in Panama was Carter, who played a major role in making the area free of the *Aedes aegypti* and *Anopheles* mosquitos. Carter organized the quarantine service of the Canal Zone and held the post of Director of Hospitals for four years.

After the findings of the Reed Commission there were other reports, notably by Hideyo Noguchi, which contested the concept that the yellow fever agent was a filtrable virus. Noguchi had isolated a slender coil-like bacterium from patients which produced a yellow fever-like illness in guinea pigs. He named it *Leptospira icteroides* which he found in Ecuador in 1919. Theiler and Sellards later identified this organism as *Leptospira icterohemorrhagicae,* the cause of Weil's disease.

The Rockefeller Foundation's International Health Division opened a yellow fever laboratory under the direction of Wilbur A. Sawyer for the express purpose of clarifying that African and South American yellow fever were the same disease. The Rockefeller Yellow Fever Commission working in Accra, Central Africa, was successful in trans-mitting the virus from a 28 year old black African with yellow fever (named Asibi) to a Rhesus monkey which had been transported from India, a country without the disease. A. H. Mahaffy and Adrian Stokes conducted these successful studies which identified a new animal host and established the existence of a huge animal reservoir. It became apparent immediately that both African monkeys and African humans possessed antibodies against the disease which indicated prior infection. Furthermore, *Aedes aegypti* was obviously not the virus' exclusive vector. Tragically, Stokes, like Lazear and others, died of yellow fever in Lagos, Nigeria, in September, 1927. Noguchi fell victim in 1928 in Accra while attempting to incriminate his leptospira as the cause of jungle yellow fever.[35]

It was now apparent that mosquitoes in the jungle canopy transmit the virus from monkey to monkey. When a non-immune person fells a tree, the infected mosquitoes which inhabit the top of trees transmit the virus to humans. This accounts for sporadic cases in Central and South America and in Central Africa even today.

Sawyer was the first to develop a yellow fever vaccine which was used successfully in laboratory workers. He and his associates used the Theiler mouse adapted French strain of yellow fever virus mixed with human immune serum. Inoculees developed antibodies but not severe reactions.

Max Theiler, patiently working first at Harvard and later at the Rockefeller Institute over many years, adapted the Asibi strain of the yellow fever virus initially to mouse brains and then to fertile hen eggs. After numerous serial passages, a remarkable biologic event of virus attentuation occurred which Theiler quickly took advantage of in 1937 by developing it into one of the world's most effective vaccines. From

1940 to 1947, the Rockefeller Foundation produced over 28 million doses of 17-D vaccine at a cost of 2.2 cents per dose. The Foundation distributed it freely to 35 different tropical countries or agencies, including the United States Army and Navy. Theiler received the Nobel Prize in 1951.[36]

The African monkey, although infected, does not die of yellow fever. Enzootic yellow fever does not normally involve man but the long-term persistence of the virus in nature does pose a threat to man, which threat depends upon varying ecological pressures which probably vary widely in different regions.

The Sudan suffered a major epidemic of about 15,000 cases in 1940, and a small, but severe, outbreak in 1959. From 1960 to 1962, Ethiopia had a sizeable epidemic. Monath listed six outbreaks between 1946 and 1970 in Nigeria in all of which the morbidity was measured in thousands and the mortality from a few to over 600.[37] In 1975, Sierra Leone, Bolivia, Colombia and Ecuador reported 130, 151, 12 and 3 cases of yellow fever, respectively. In 1976, Brazil and Ecuador reported 15 and 45 cases, respectively, with sporadic case reports from Africa and South America.[38]

Summary

Based upon clinical and epidemiologic data, two Marylanders, Potter and Davidge, were among the first to disagree with Rush and his contagion theory; they told him so and published their views. To prove this point, Potter went to the extreme of inoculating himself with presumedly infected material. Stubbins Ffirth, a young University of Pennsylvania medical student, did the same four years later. Rush ultimately abandoned his originally held views.

Crawford, of Baltimore, although not the originator of the insect concept of transmission of infectious agents, published his concepts in 1811. Josiah Nott of Mobile, Alabama, in 1848 suggested an insect origin of yellow fever, including mosquitoes.

In 1898, Carter clearly noted that, after identification of an index case of yellow fever, an extrinsic incubation period was necessary before the evolution of secondary cases.

Walter Reed, James Carroll, and Lazear and Agramonte, helped prove Finlay's original concept that the *Aedes aegypti* mosquito was the natural vector of yellow fever. Carroll himself was the first experimentally induced case.

After the findings of the Reed Commission, further laboratory studies led to the isolation of the virus and the development of an effective vaccine. However, further studies indicate that mosquitoes in the jungle transmit the virus from monkey to monkey, which do not die from the disease. The persistence of the virus in nature poses a continuous threat to man and epidemics continue to occur.

Notes

1. H. A. Kelley, *Walter Reed and Yellow Fever* (New York: McClure Phillips, 1906), p. 89.

2. James Carroll, "Remarks on the history, cause and mode of transmission of yellow fever," *J. Assoc. Military Surgeons of U.S.A.,* 1903, *13:* 177-210, 232-244; p. 199.

3. G. W. Corner, *The Autobiography of Benjamin Rush* (Philadelphia: Publ. by the American Philosophical Society by Princeton University Press, 1951).

4. Cited by Eugene S. Ferguson, *Truxtun of the Constellation* (Baltimore: The Johns Hopkins Press, 1956); Kent Porter, "The birth of the Constellation: Troubled waters and triumph," *Baltimore Sun Magazine,* Sept. 7, 1975; Walter Lord, Personal communication.

5. David M. Reese, *Observations on the Epidemic of 1819 as it Prevailed in a Part of the City of Baltimore* (Baltimore: John D. Troy, 1819), p. 89.

6. Ibid.

7. A. Smith, *Yellow Fever in Galveston* (Austin: University of Texas Press, 1951), p. 95; Benjamin Rush, *Medical Inquiries and Observations,* 3rd ed. (Philadelphia: Benjamin & Thomas Kite [etc.], 1809), vol. 4, p. 238.

8. Reese, *Observations on the Epidemic of 1819,* p. ii.

9. Nathaniel Potter, *A Memoir of Contagion, More Especially as It Respects the Yellow Fever.* Read in Convention of the Medical and Chirurgical of Maryland, June 1817 (Baltimore: Edward J. Coale, 1818), p. ii.

10. Ibid., p. iii.

11. Ibid., p. 113.

12. Ibid., p. 52.

13. John B. Davidge, *A Treatise on the Autumnal Endemial Epidemic of Tropical Climates, Commonly Called Yellow Fever, Containing Its Origin, History, Nature and Cure, together with a Few Reflections on the Proximate Cause of Diseases* (Baltimore: William Warner, 1813; first published in 1798).

14. Kelly, *Walter Reed,* p. 278; Potter, *Memoir of Contagion,* p. 53.

15. Kelly, *Walter Reed,* p. 87; Jean Devèse, *An Inquiry into and Observations upon the Causes and Effects of the Epidemic Which Raged in Philadelphia from the Month of August till the Middle of December, 1793* (Philadelphia, 1794).

16. Thomas Drysdale, "Letters written by Dr. Drysdale to Dr. Benjamin Rush giving an account of the yellow fever in Baltimore, 1794," *Phila. Med. Museum,* 1794, 22-121, 241-261; James Carroll, "Remarks on the epidemic of yellow fever in Baltimore," *Old Maryland,* Feb. 1906, *2* (2).

17. John Crawford, *A Lecture, Introductory to a Course of Lectures in the Cause, Seat and Cure of Diseases* (Baltimore: Edward J. Coale, 1811), p. 49.

18. Ibid., p. 37; R. La Roche, *Yellow Fever Considered in Its Historical, Pathological, Etiological and Therapeutic Relations* (Philadelphia, 1855).

19. H. N. Simpson, "The impact of disease on American history," *New England J. Med.,* 1954, *250:* 697; J. H. Rose, *Life of Napoleon* (London: G. Bell & Son, 1913), 2 vol., p. 1018; Alistair Cooke, *America* (New York: Alfred A. Knopf, 1974).

20. Josiah H. Nott, "Essay on yellow fever," *New Orleans Med. & Surg. J.,* 1900, *52:* 617-636.

21. H. R. Carter, "Are vessels infected with yellow fever? Some personal observations," *Med. Record,* 1902, *61:* 441-444.

22. H. R. Carter, "Note on interval between infecting and secondary cases of yellow fever from records at Orwood and Taylor, Miss., in 1898," *New Orleans Med. &. Surg. J.,* 1900, *52:* 617-636.

23. Ibid.

24. E. D. Richter, "Henry Rose Carter, an overlooked skeptical epidemiologist," *New Eng. J. Med.,* 1967, *277:* 734-738.

25. National Library of Medicine: Papers, Letters, Manuscripts relating to H. R. Carter, Letter of February 26, 1902 (cited by Richter vet 21).

26. Richter, "Henry Rose Carter," p. 737.

27. Kelly, Walter Reed; J. Carroll, "A brief review of the etiology of yellow fever," *New York Med. J. and Philadelphia Med. J., combined,* 1904, *79:* 241-245, 307-310; p. 245.

28. G. M. Sternberg, Address presented to the Johns Hopkins Historical Club Meeting, October 14, 1907. Held in memory of Major James Carroll, M.D., U.S.A., *Bull. Johns Hopkins Hosp.,* 1908, *19:* 8.

29. For the contribution of this and other original letters of Walter Reed and James Carroll to the University of Maryland School of Medicine, the author expresses grateful appreciation to Mrs. Carolyn Carroll Buehler, daughter of Dr. Carroll, and Mr. George D. Buehler and Mrs. Carolyn Morris, his grandchildren.

30. Albert E. Truby, *Memoir of Walter Reed* (New York & London: Paul B. Hoeber, 1943), p. 75.

31. Kelly, *Walter Reed and Yellow Fever,* p. 164.

32. Ibid., p. 270, 271.

33. Ibid., p. 271; Carroll, "Brief review of the etiology of yellow fever."

34. From a collection of Reed and Carroll letters, University of Maryland.

35. Greer Williams, *Virus Hunters* (New York: Alfred A. Knopf, 1959).

36. Ibid., p. 175.

37. T. P. Monath, Cah. O.R.S.T.O.M., *Ser. Ent. Med. Parasitol.,* 1972, pp. 10, 169.

38. *World Health Reports,* 30, no. 2, Geneva, 1977.

Discussion

Saul Jarcho

Some Ancient and Medieval Statements about Fever

In antiquity the fevers were a highly disorderly area of medical knowledge—at least as disorderly as anything else. This is shown by the headings *febris* and *febres* in the Latin index which fills volume XX of Kühn's *Galen*.[1] If the 12 preliminary columns (pp. 248-253) on the general characteristics and causes of the fevers are disregarded, the reader comes to 19 columns (pp. 254-263) which deal with individual fevers, arranged alphabetically from *febris acmastica* to *febris vapida* and *febres vehementes*. In this listing of individual fevers and traits there are approximately 77 discrete entries. Some of the more important are as follows:

ardens	hecticae	quotidianae
biliosa	intermittentes	semitertiana
causi	malignae	synochus
contentes	pestilens	tertiana
continus	putridae	typhodes
diariae (s. ephemerae)	quartanae	vehementes

To view this list as disorder is an unjustifiable retrojection of contemporary concepts into the past. Let us regard it instead as evidence of an earlier kind of order, in which entities are named by single traits and in which most entities show little distinct relation to others. Later attempts to introduce order into the subject are exemplified by the *Nosologia media* of François Boissier de Sauvages (1768) and by the writings of other eighteenth-century nosologic taxonomists.

The ancient disorder and the difficult nosologies of later times are especially impressive because we have come to feel that the subject of fevers is one of the *most* susceptible to orderly presentation.

132

Numerous passages in Galen allow us to understand the Greek concept of fever as an increase in natural heat accompanied by frequency and intensity of the pulse.[2] The heat usually affected the whole body but on occasion was only local.[3] Whereas older physicians had considered fever to be a disease *per se,* Erasistratus and several other newcomers had considered it a symptom;[4] this statement indicates an evolution of the concept. In a famous passage in the *Timaeus* Plato[5] mentions quotidian, tertian, and quartan fevers, and even notes the obstinacy of the quartan. It is interesting that the Latins used the terms *algere* and *aestuare,* to feel cold and to feel hot (subjectively), as distinct from *frigere* and *calere,* to be cold and to be hot (objectively).[6] Avicenna in his elaborate systematic discussion of fevers mentions a kind called *lipyria,* in which the heat is concealed and only cold is apparent.[7] The heat was internal.

Evolution of the Concept of Certain Individual Fevers

In any study of the history of the fevers it soon becomes evident that our concepts of individual febrile diseases have undergone considerable evolution. Excellent examples of this are typhus, malaria and yellow fever.

Typhus. We start with the old concept of typhus as a continued fever accompanied by clouding of the mind. The Hippocratic treatise *De morbis internis* describes five kinds or examples of typhus.[8] The term was also used vaguely for continued or severe fevers, whether or not mental obnubilation was present, e.g. *typhus icterodes* was one name (used in later times) for yellow fever.

A major advance was the differentiation of typhoid from typhus by W. W. Gerhard[9] in 1837, resulting from the combined study of clinical medicine and morbid anatomy. It illustrates, also, the value of travel, Gerhard having studied in Europe as well as in America. Perhaps the ancient tradition of the wandering scientist or the medieval tradition of the itinerant scholar should receive some of the credit.

An important later stage in the concept of typhus-like fevers was the distinct separation of paratyphoid fever by Achard and Bensaude in 1896.[10] This was a contribution of the Golden Age of Bacteriology.

Late nineteenth-century concepts and their antecedents are revealed by the terminology used in Germany, Russia, and England. Toward the end of the century it was usual to distinguish three kinds of typhus:

I. *Typhus abdominalis*
    Germany: Bauchtyphus
    Russia: brushnoy tif
    England: typhoid fever
II. *Typhus petechialis*
    Germany: Flecktyphus
    Russia: sipnoy tif
    England: typhus
III. *Typhus recurrens*
    Germany: febris recurrens; recurrens[11]
    Russia: vozvratny tif
    England: relapsing fever

Later developments were the differentiation of typhus into louse-borne epidemic typhus and flea-borne murine typhus; the recognition of long-delayed recurrence (Brill's disease); and the segregation of tick-borne and mite-borne rickettsioses such as Rocky Mountain spotted fever and tsutsugamushi. Even nowadays some of the Oriental rickettsioses are occasionally referred to as scrub typhus.

We now possess an entire subtaxonomy of rickettsioses. The principal factor which made possible the differentiation of the concept of typhus into an orderly taxonomy of increasingly well-characterized entities has been the developments in bacteriology and virology, assisted by serology, immunology, and entomology.

Malaria. The ancient concept of what we now call malaria was that of fever and chills. The fever was periodic; cyclic recurrence—quotidian, tertian, and quartan—was well known.[12] There was no dependable way of distinguishing such cases from the recurring fever and chills that might occur in other diseases, except that fever and chills happening in the presence of an obvious focus, such as osteomyelitis or puerperal sepsis, were easy to identify.

As with typhus, some of the conceptual evolution is reflected in the terminology.[13] The term *mal'aria* is recorded in Italian in 1560 and signifies not only bad air but implies pathogenicity, i.e. the bad air is not only malodorous but is a cause of febrile sickness. As is well known, the term *mal'aria*, with no alteration in spelling, entered the English literature in 1740 through the agency of Horace Walpole. The apostrophe later was lost and the two Italian words became fused into the single English word *malaria.* It is important to remember that throughout almost the whole of the nineteenth century the English word *malaria* was not the name of a disease; it was the name of a miasm or vapor, usually malodorous, that caused disease. At that stage of conceptual evolution the diseases that were caused by malaria had numerous names, e.g. autumnal fever and intermittent fever.

With the discovery made by Laveran—an example of the benefits of imperialism, colonialism, and militarism—the old and excessively simple concept of intermittent fever caused by miasm was forced to give way.[14] Concomitantly the terminology was also forced to change: the term *malarial fever,* a fever caused by bad air, began to change to the simple designation *malaria,* a febrile disease caused by plasmodia. This transition can be seen in the first edition of Osler's textbook of medicine (1893), which was written at a time when Laveran's discovery had been confirmed by numerous observers but had not yet won full acceptance.

The increase in the number of recognized plasmodial pathogens of man from one to three—increased to four by the addition of *Plasmodium ovale*—did not alter the concept that is denoted by the word malaria, nor was the concept altered by the important later discovery of the exo-erythrocytic stages of the plasmodia. The discovery of the plasmodia however can be said to have given the concept of malaria increased precision because it made possible the differentiation between malaria and other tropical and subtropical fevers such as kala-azar and brucellosis.

Yellow fever. The best available evidence, not universally accepted,[15] indicates that while yellow fever may have been epidemic or endemic in Mexico before that area became known to Europeans, the disease was absent from Europe, Africa and the Orient before the Europeans entered Mexico in the early sixteenth century. While this is probably true, it is obvious that cases of jaundice occurring in the presence of fever (but *not* caused by yellow fever) must have been observed in antiquity and in the Middle Ages. To exclude these from consideration is to simplify the record unjustifiably. The numerous fevers mentioned by Galen include a *febris auriginosa,* in which a color similar to that of icterus was produced, the liver was enlarged, and the skin became dirty and yellow.[16] Avicenna speaks of fever concurrent with jaundice in the presence of an abscess.[17]

Numerous outbreaks of yellow fever were recorded in the late seventeenth and early eighteenth century, but Fielding Garrison[18] could trace the term "yellow fever" no farther back than 1750. Under the year of 1748 the *Oxford English Dictionary*[19] cites John Lining as having stated that the term was in use in America. Benjamin Franklin used the expression in 1744[20] and Francisco Guerra's *American Medical Bibliography*[21] records the use of the term in two newspapers dated 1739.

The chief health officer of a neighboring republic has told me that in at least one West Indian Island there are early tombstones marked YELLOW FEVER. These promising epigraphic sources are now being investigated, but the results are not yet available and the dates have not been reported.

In the eighteenth century the expression "yellow fever" referred to cases of fever accompanied by jaundice and vomiting, the infection showing usually (but not always) a marked epidemic tendency, a brief course, and a high case fatality rate. It has been established that Benjamin Rush's concept of yellow fever was based on cases recorded in a manuscript of John Mitchell and that these were probably instances of sporadic infectious hepatitis, not yellow fever. Mitchell's patients were treated between 1737 and 1742.[22]

During the eighteenth, nineteenth, and early twentieth centuries the concept of yellow fever and also the diagnosis in individual cases was complicated by confusion with other diseases, especially with what we now call malaria, typhoid fever, and infectious hepatitis. For example La Roche discusses in detail the question of whether yellow fever is a continued, a remittent, or an intermittent fever.[23] In a special section of his *Handbook of Geographical and Historical Pathology*[24] August Hirsch presents information about 34 outbreaks of jaundice, mainly European, which occurred between 1745 and 1884. Could any of these have been examples of yellow fever? Hirsch says that often "the malady ran the course of a simple catarrhal icterus."

A more striking example of the difficulties occurs in the writings of Armand Trousseau, one of the greatest physicians who ever lived. In one of his lectures he said: "in upwards of a thousand yellow fever patients who came under my observation, not one had jaundice."[25] Whether these were cases of dengue or mild yellow fever or some other infection cannot be determined without additional investigation, since no details are given. As Dr. Wilbur Downs has written,[26] the fact that mild cases of yellow fever exist and may preponderate in an outbreak was demonstrated by Josiah Nott in the nineteenth century. Dr. Downs has pointed out, further,[27] that "physicians to-day, overlooking Nott's admonitions and the admonitions of later writers, cherish a concept of the 'classical yellow fever case' . . . yet when they see such a case out of epidemic context they are likely to call it anything but yellow fever. Even less likely is the possibility of correct diagnosis where fever is mild in the occasional case. . . ."

Some later phases and later vicissitudes in the elucidation of infectious fevers accompanied by jaundice are exemplified by Weil's work on leptospirosis,[28] the erroneous work of Noguchi, the discovery of jungle yellow fever,[29] and the recent research on the differentiation and subdivision of what is now called infectious hepatitis,[30] a complex of at least three entities.

As we study the changes in concepts, whether of typhus, or malaria, or yellow fever, it becomes apparent that the major developmental impulse has been the discovery of the causes, as revealed by bacteriology and virology. Our most satisfying taxonomy is therefore based on etiology. The etiology once secured, the entire epidemiological, ecological, and human picture can then be clarified.

Notes

1. C. G. Kühn, editor, *Claudii Galeni Opera omnia* (Leipzig: Cnobloch, 1821-33; reprographic edition Hildesheim: Olms, 1946). Two of the best places for a medical historian to play hooky are the index to Kühn's *Galen* and the *Index-Catalogue of the Library of the Surgeon General's Office.*

2. Several definitions are given in Galen's *Definitiones medicae* CLXXXV (Kühn XIX, 398). See also *De morborum causes* II (Kühn VII, 4).

3. *De causes pulsuum* IV (Kühn IX, 165); *De morborum differentiis* V (Kühn VI, 849).

4. Galen, *Introductio seu medicus* XIII (Kühn XIV, 729).

5. Plato, *Timaeus* 86 A.

6. C. T. Lewis and C. Short, *A Latin Dictionary* (Oxford: Clarendon Press, 1879; reprinted 1969), p. 83.

7. Avicenna, *Canon*, Book IV, Fen I, Tract II, Chap. L.

8. Hippocrates, *Oeuvres complètes.* Ed. and trans. E. Littré (Paris, 1839-61), VII, 260-265.

9. W. W. Gerhard, *Amer. J. Med. Sci.*, 1837, *20:* 289-322.

10. E. C. Achard and R. Bensaude, "Infections paratyphoïdiques," *Bull. Soc. Méd. Hôp. Paris*, ser. 3, 1896, *13:* 820-833.

11. German authors usually wrote *febris recurrena* or *recurrens.* The terms *typhus recurrens, Rückfallstyphus,* and *wiederkehrende Fieber* were also used and are to be found in the *Index Catalogue,* ser. 1, vol. 4, p. 768.

12. Readers of Shakespeare will remember Mistress Quickly's malapropism ("Sir John . . . is so shaked of a burning quotidian tertian, that it is most lamentable to behold"), *King Henry V,* II. 1. 115.

13. Saul Jarcho, "A cartographic and literary study of the word *malaria,*"*J. Hist. Med.,* 1970, *25:* 31-39.

14. Charles-Louis-Alphonse Laveran, "Un nouveau parasite trouvé dans le sang de plusieurs malades atteinte de fievre palustre," *Bull. Soc. méd. Hôp. Paris (Mém.),* 2e sér., 1881, *17:* 158-164.

15. Findlay advocated an African origin. See G. M. Findlay, "The first recognized epidemic of yellow fever," *Trans. Roy. Soc. Trop Med. & Hyg.,* 1941, *35:* 143-154.

16. Galen, *Definitiones medicae* 193 (Kühn XIX, 400).

17. Avicenna, *Canon,* Book IV, Fen I, Treatise II, Chap. VII.

18. Fielding H. Garrison, *An Introduction to the History of Medicine.* 4th ed. (Philadelphia: Saunders, 1929), p. 404.

19. *The Compact Edition of the Oxford English Dictionary* (New York: Oxford University Press, 1971; reprinted 1975), p. 3855.

20. B. Franklin, "Letter to Cadwallader Colden, Oct. 25, 1744," *The Letters and Papers of Cadwallader Colden* (New York: New York Historical Society), vol. 3, pp. 77-78.

21. Francisco Guerra, *American Medical Bibliography,* 1639-1783 (New York: Lathrop Harper, 1962). See p. 441 (*Boston Evening-Post,* Feb. 19, 1739) and p. 477 (*Boston Weekly Post-Boy,* Jan. 22, 1739). See also a letter of Benjamin Franklin to Cadwallader Colden, Oct. 25, 1744 (*The Letters and Papers of Cadwallader Colden,* vol. 3, pp. 76-77).

22. Saul Jarcho, "John Mitchell, Benjamin Rush, and Yellow Fever," *Bull. Hist. Med.,* 1957, *31:* 132-136.

23. L. La Roche, *Yellow Fever* (Philadelphia: Blanchard & Lea, 1855), vol. 1, p. 426-437; see esp. p. 436, also p. 560 and pp. 579-580.

24. August Hirsch, *Handbook of Geographical and Historical Pathology* (London: Sydenham Society, 1883-86), vol 3, pp. 417-425.

25. A. Trousseau, *Lectures on Clinical Medicine Delivered at the Hôtel-Dieu,* Paris (London: New Sydenham Society, 1867-82), vol. 4, p. 321.

26. W. G. Downs, "Yellow fever and Josiah Clark Nott," *Bull. N. Y. Acad. Med.,* 1974, *50:* 499-508; see p. 501.

27. Ibid., p. 502.

28. A. Weill, "Ueber eine eigenthümliche, mit Milztumor, Icterus und Nephrisit einhergehende, acute Infectionskrankheit," *Deutsche Arch. f. klin. Med.,* 1886, *39:* 209-232.

29. F. L. Soper and others, "Yellow fever without *Aëdes Aegypti.* Study of a rural epidemic in the Valle do Chanaan, Espirito Santo, Brazil, 1932," *Amer. J. Hyg.,* 1933, *18:* 555-587.

30. S. Krugman, J. P. Giles, and J. Hammond, "Infectious hepatitis. Evidence for two distinctive clinical, epidemiological, and immunological types of infection," *J.A.M.A.,* 1967, *200:* 365-373.

Contributors

William G. Cochran, M.A., LL.D., Emeritus Professor of Statistics, Harvard University (deceased)

Alfred S. Evans, M.D., M.P.H., Department of Epidemiology and Public Health, Yale University School of Medicine, 333 Cedar St., New Haven, Conn., 06510

John M. Eyler, Ph.D., Department of the History of Medicine and Biological Sciences, Diehl Hall, University of Minnesota, Minneapolis, Minn. 55455

Caroline Hannaway, Ph.D., The Johns Hopkins University, Institute of the History of Medicine, 1900 E. Monument St., Baltimore, Md. 21205

Donald A. Henderson, M.D., M.P.H., The Johns Hopkins University, School of Hygiene and Public Health, 615 N. Wolfe St., Baltimore, Md. 21205

Victor L. Hilts, Ph.D., Department of History of Science, South Hall, University of Wisconsin, Madison, Wis. 53706

Saul Jarcho, M.D., Consulting Editor-in-Chief, *Transactions and Studies of the College of Physicians of Philadelphia.* 35 East 85th St., New York, N.Y. 10028

Alexander Langmuir, M.D., M.P.H., Department of Preventive Medicine, Harvard Medical School, Boston, Mass. 02115

Abraham M. Lilienfeld, M.D., M.P.H., Department of Epidemiology, The Johns Hopkins University, School of Hygiene and Public Health, 615 N. Wolfe St., Baltimore, Md. 21205

David E. Lilienfeld, M.S.E., Faculty of Engineering, The Johns Hopkins University. 3501 St. Paul St., Baltimore, Md. 21218

Genevieve Miller, Ph.D., Retired Director, Howard Dittrick Museum of Historical Medicine. The Johns Hopkins University, Institute of the History of Medicine, 1900 E. Monument St., Baltimore, Md. 21205

Peter H. Niebyl, M.D., Ph.D., The Johns Hopkins University, Institute of the History of Medicine, 1900 E. Monument St., Baltimore, Md. 21205

Phyllis A. Richmond, Ph.D., M.L.S., Case-Western Reserve University, 109 Euclid Ave., Cleveland, Ohio 44106

Daphne A. Roe, M.D., Division of Nutritional Sciences, Cornell University, Ithaca, N.Y. 14853

Theodore E. Woodward, M.D., Department of Medicine, University of Maryland, School of Medicine, Baltimore, Md. 21201

Index

141